ENT OSCEs

Revised and expanded for the third edition, this book is both a guide for your first ENT job and a tried and tested revision guide covering all aspects of the MRCS (ENT) objective structured clinical examination (OSCE). Written by a team of ENT specialists, the accessible text follows a step-by-step approach with each OSCE station based on the style of past exam questions. Recent changes to the structure of the examination, including those during COVID and post-COVID are included.

With over 120 colour images, the guide remains unrivalled as a tool with which to prepare for ENT exams. It is essential reading for candidates of the MRCS (ENT) OSCE and will also aid trainees in preparation for specialty registrar national selection interviews. It is highly recommended for GPs wishing to refresh their knowledge of how to assess common ENT problems and will also be an ideal reference for any junior doctor learning to take histories and examinations in their first ENT post. Equally, it is an invaluable resource for medical students undertaking their ENT attachment and in preparation for final examinations.

MasterPass Series

For more information about this series please visit: https://www.routledge.com/MasterPass/book-series/CRCMASPASS

ENT OSCEs: A Guide to your first ENT job and passing the MRCS (ENT) OSCE

Third Edition

Peter Kullar
Joseph Manjaly
Livy Kenyon

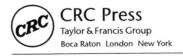

CRC Press
Taylor & Francis Group
Boca Raton London New York

CRC Press is an imprint of the
Taylor & Francis Group, an **informa** business

Third edition published 2023
by CRC Press
6000 Broken Sound Parkway NW, Suite 300, Boca Raton, FL 33487-2742

and by CRC Press
4 Park Square, Milton Park, Abingdon, Oxon, OX14 4RN

CRC Press is an imprint of Taylor & Francis Group, LLC

© 2023 Taylor & Francis Group, LLC

ISBN: 9781032209807 (hbk)
ISBN: 9781032191737 (pbk)
ISBN: 9781003266204 (ebk)

DOI: 10.1201/b23029

Typeset in Palatino
by KnowledgeWorks Global Ltd.

Contents

Contents

Foreword

Exams are a 'necessary evil' in life. As surgeons we have exposure to more than our fair share of these 'evils' leaving many of us with a lifelong sense of deep foreboding whenever we cross the portals of the Royal College of Surgeons! However, the tools to help one successfully negotiate these life events are becoming more and more effective. This excellent book, now in its highly successful third edition, exposes the reader not just to the type and style of questions likely to be encountered in the OSCE sections of the MRCS (ENT) exams but also gives advice on practical preparation, and how to make these situations less daunting.

All exams have a syllabus and whilst there is no short cut to the acquisition of knowledge to satisfy that syllabus, knowledge alone is not sufficient to guarantee a pass. Exam technique plays an enormous part, particularly in relation to OSCE and communication skills stations. Reading and re-reading this book will equip the candidate with the best chance to avoid the dreaded 'See you again in four months'! The scenarios set out in this well illustrated book are the sorts of cases likely to be encountered on a regular basis in any busy ENT department. The distillation of this knowledge will therefore not just help one to pass the formal exams but also to become a better clinician.

It's a pleasure to provide the foreword to the third edition of this text – one that has now provided countless current registrars and consultants in the UK and internationally a guided way to MRCS. On a personal note, I had the pleasure of being Joe Manjaly's trainer and he is now my consultant colleague at the Royal National ENT Hospital. He is a wonderful and inspirational teacher and I look forward to his continued and ever-increasing contribution to the ENT world.

Jeremy Lavy
FRCS (Eng) FRCS (ORL-HNS)
Consultant ENT Surgeon
The Royal National ENT Hospital & University College London Hospitals, UK

Preface to the Third Edition

The beginnings of this book were born back in 2011 when we met on a DOHNS preparation course and together realised there was a need for a revision textbook, as there was no such resource available at the time. Over ten years later, we are delighted that this book has been so well received by trainees, and it gives us great encouragement whenever we meet a colleague who tells us he or she has our book and that it made a difference to his or her preparation.

Ali Carter and Richard Fox helped us bring out a fresh updated version in 2016, and it's crucial to continue keeping relevant and up to date for the exam, for which we are grateful to Livy Kenyon who joins the authorship for this third edition.

One of us is a consultant now, and in the years since the first edition, it has brought great satisfaction seeing many trainees come through the ranks assisted by these books to go on and make great contributions to the ENT community.

We trust this new, updated edition of our book will continue to maintain its place as an endorsed text by trainees taking the Diploma of Otolaryngology – Head and Neck Surgery (DO-HNS)/MRCS (ENT) exam, as well as those preparing for Specialty Training Year 3 national selection.

Many trainees comment that the histories and examinations sections of this book are equally useful to those in other training grades learning to do an ENT clinic for the first time. Once you've passed your exam, do consider lending your copy to your newest Foundation/General Practice Trainee although also bear in mind that some trainees still come back to this book when starting to prepare for FCRS (ORL-HNS)!

Joe Manjaly and Peter Kullar
January 2022

Acknowledgements

Thank you to our friends and colleagues for contributions in this book:

Major Contributors and Chapter Authors:

Alison Carter
ENT Specialty Registrar
London Deanery North Thames rotation, UK

Richard Fox
ENT Registrar, Sydney, Australia

Philip Yates
Freeman Hospital, Newcastle-upon-Tyne, UK

Additional Contributors:

Deepak Chandrasekharan
ENT Specialty Registrar
London Deanery North Thames rotation, UK

Manish George
ENT Specialty Registrar
London Deanery North Thames rotation, UK

Andrew Hall
Consultant ENT Surgeon
University Hospital of Wales & Noah's Ark Children's Hospital for Wales, UK

Nora Haloob
ENT Specialty Registrar
London Deanery North Thames rotation, UK

John Hardman
ENT Specialty Registrar
London Deanery North Thames rotation, UK

Samantha Holmes
Clinical Lead Head & Neck Speech & Language Therapist
Oxford University Hospitals, UK

Fiona McClenaghan
ENT Specialty Registrar
London Deanery North Thames rotation, UK

Robert Nash
Consultant ENT Surgeon
Great Ormond Street Hospital, London UK

Authors

Peter Kullar is an Academic Clinical Lecturer and Cochlear Implant and Otology fellow at Cambridge University Hospitals and obtained FRCS (HNS-ORL) in 2021. He graduated from Cambridge University and successfully obtained a PhD in Clinical Neurosciences focussing on the mechanisms of mitochondrial hearing loss.

Joseph Manjaly is a Consultant ENT Surgeon at the Royal National ENT Hospital and University College London Hospitals, specialising in Otology and Auditory Implant surgery for adults and children. He completed higher surgical training in the London North Thames region followed by an advanced fellowship in otology and hearing implantation at Cambridge University Hospitals. He has been involved in teaching since his undergraduate years at Bristol University and has co-authored a number of trainee textbooks widely used in the UK and abroad. He has been actively involved in training issues regionally and nationally, holding a number of committee roles and teaching on a number of national courses.

Livy Kenyon is a specialty registrar in the Thames Valley ENT rotation, working at the Royal Berkshire Hospital. She graduated from Cambridge University and continued her Foundation and Core training in East of England. She was awarded the Membership of the Royal College of Surgeons (Ear, Nose and Throat) at the beginning of her Core Surgical Training in 2018 and has mentored junior colleagues through the exam since. She has been involved with supervision and teaching since being a clinical supervisor during medical school, as well as during her year as a junior anatomy demonstrator at Cambridge University, where she was an undergraduate supervisor in head and neck anatomy and founded a DOHNS anatomy revision course.

Abbreviations

ACE	angiotensin-converting enzyme
ANCA	anti-neutrophil cytoplasmic antibody
AOAE	sautomated otoacoustic emissions
AOM	acute otitis media
AOT	Association of Otolaryngologists in Training
BIPP	bismuth, iodoform and paraffin paste
BPPV	benign paroxysmal positional vertigo
CBT	cognitive behavioural therapy
CNS	central nervous system
CSC	Churg–Strauss syndrome
CSF	cerebrospinal fluid
CSOM	chronic suppurative otitis media
CT	computed tomography
CXR	chest X-ray
DO-HNS	Diploma of Otolaryngology – Head and Neck Surgery
EAC	external auditory canal
ENT	ear, nose and throat
ESR	erythrocyte sedimentation rate
FBC	full blood count
FNA	fine needle aspiration
FNE	flexible nasendoscopy
FOSIT	feeling of something in the throat
FY	Foundation Year
GP	general practitioner
GPVTS	General Practice Vocational Training Scheme
GRBAS	grade, roughness, breathiness, asthenia, strain scale
HIV	human immunodeficiency virus
ICP	intracranial pressure

INR	international normalised ratio
JVP	jugular venous pulse
LMN	lower motor neuron
LPR	laryngopharyngeal reflux
MRCS	Membership of the Royal College of Surgeons
MRI	magnetic resonance imaging
OD	olfactory dysfunction
OE	otitis externa
OME	otitis media with effusion
OSCE	objective structured clinical examination
PNS	post-nasal space
PPI	proton-pump inhibitor
PTA	pure-tone audiometry
SCC	squamous cell carcinoma
SHO	senior house officer
SNHL	sensorineural hearing loss
ST3	Specialty Training Year 3
TB	tuberculosis
TM	tympanic membrane
TORCH	toxoplasmosis, other, rubella, cytomegalovirus, herpes simplex virus
U+E	surea and electrolytes
UMN	upper motor neuron
URTI	upper respiratory tract infection
USS	ultrasound scan
WG	Wegener granulomatosis

The DO-HNS and MRCS (ENT) Examination and How to Pass It

The Diploma of Otolaryngology – Head and Neck Surgery (DO-HNS) has existed in one form or another since 2003, after replacing the old Diploma of Laryngology and Otology. Your reason for sitting the examination will most likely be as a route into higher ear, nose and throat (ENT) training or as a way of showing a special interest as part of general practice or allied specialty training. DO-HNS in combination with Membership of the Royal College of Surgeons (MRCS), or the 'MRCS (ENT)', is a requirement in order to be eligible to attend the ENT national selection interviews for registrar training, although it is not required to be passed at the time of application.

The examination consists of two parts: Part 1, a 2-hour written paper comprising multiple-choice questions and extended matching questions, and Part 2, the objective structured clinical examination (OSCE) on which this book focuses. Historically, candidates for ENT Specialty Training Year 3 (ST3) tended to sit the full DO-HNS examination in addition to both parts of the regular MRCS examination.

In May 2011, 'MRCS (ENT)' was introduced and was awarded to candidates passing MRCS Part A and the DO-HNS OSCE. The DO-HNS examination, until September 2021 could still be sat as a stand-alone examination for those outside of ENT higher surgical training, most commonly, but not exclusively, general practitioners (GPs), or for prospective ENT trainees who wished to complete it alongside the traditional MRCS sat by other surgical specialties. From February 2022 the DOHNS OSCE has been renamed the MRCS ENT OSCE. Those candidates who pass MRCS Part A and MRCS ENT OSCE will be eligible for MRCS (ENT). In addition, candidates who have passed DOHNS part A before it was discontinued and the MRCS ENT OSCE will still be eligible for the DOHNS diploma.

It is important to note that when applying for ENT national selection, there are no additional points awarded for either combination; therefore, the choice is a personal one for each prospective candidate. Be sure to get up to speed with the latest examination announcements and the core syllabus on the DO-HNS website (http://www.intercollegiatemrcsexams.org.uk/dohns). We are confident that using this book will provide a firm grounding for passing the OSCE. Whilst there is no rule governing experience, time spent in an ENT job is invaluable, as many of the questions are designed to test 'on-the-job experience'.

The examination is held three times per year, rotating among London, Edinburgh, Glasgow and Dublin, so be sure to register and pay fees in good time. The colleges are very strict on application deadlines and they tend not to make exceptions for late entries. It is a good idea to sort out travel and accommodation as early as possible, as the later these details are arranged, the more expensive they become. You will also need to make sure you have appropriate cover in place and have swapped on-calls as, if you happen to be taking the exam at a distant location, you often will need 2 days in order to get there and back, and you may not know your specific exam date within the given window until after the 6 weeks required notice period most hospitals have in place for leave requests.

Allow 2–3 months' preparation time alongside your normal clinical commitments. In addition to this book, you will find it useful to work through an ENT picture atlas and to selectively read a more comprehensive ENT textbook, of which there are many on the market.

The importance of the communication skills section of the examination must be stressed, and many candidates tend to find this section problematic. For those who are not native English speakers or do not have a degree from a UK medical school, it may be appropriate to consider further training in communication skills. Most importantly, you must practise the examination and communication scenarios *ad nauseam*. In our experience, obliging friends and relatives are a great source of practice. It may also be worthwhile attending a dedicated DO-HNS revision course. It is surprising how effectively a substantial financial outlay focuses the revision-weary mind.

You will find that the examination question style is similar to those in this book. At the time of writing, the OSCE consists of around 25 stations plus three to four rest stations, each lasting 7 minutes. Approximately 20 of these stations are unmanned written stations. The examination lasts approximately 3½ hours, but with the added administration time it allows at least 6 hours door to door.

It is also important to note that the mark scheme for the written stations tends to accept short, succinct answers. Largely, time is in abundance for these stations. Do not feel you have to write long paragraphs. Often, a sentence or a few words will be enough to secure the marks. In our experience, for each question the number of lines given in the answer booklet corresponds with the number of marks available. For example, a question with four lines in the answer space means there are four possible marks to be picked up. We cannot stress enough how important it is that you read and re-read the question. It sounds obvious, but make sure you actually answer the question. For example, if the question asks for four causes of something, you will be scored only for the first four that you list. This means if you list six causes and the first two are wrong, you will only score two marks, even if the next four are correct.

Be reassured that pass rates have tended to be between 45% and 75% in recent years. With some considered preparation this is an eminently passable and fair examination.

On a final note, as you can imagine, a 3½ hour examination is long and most certainly feels it. It is important to be rested before the examination. Some people find it useful to take a small snack with them to keep up those flagging blood sugar levels.

Joseph Manjaly and Peter Kullar

General Tips for the Communication and History Stations

The communication stations are probably the most intimidating part of the examination. You are faced with an actor and an examiner. To those not familiar with the OSCE set-up this can be daunting. Staying calm and unflustered will be to your advantage. Be assured that there are plenty of marks available for the simple things. It is vital to ignore the contrived nature of the situation and treat the actor as a patient, as you would in clinical practice. Do not expect too much interaction from the examiner; it is normal for the examiner to remain entirely passive. This can be a little disconcerting if you are looking for affirmation. Likewise, do not rely on the examiner for timekeeping. There will be no signal that the 7 minutes allotted for the station is coming to an end. It is well worth practising some of the scenarios in this book, to give you an idea of how best to manage the time effectively.

For all of the history stations it is useful to adopt the 'open to closed' question approach. Start general and then work on to the specifics of the presenting complaint. A useful general opener could be: 'Could you explain to me in your own words the symptoms that you have been experiencing?'

It is also useful to contextualise the patient's symptoms, so ask early on in the consultation about the effect of the symptoms on the patient's life. This is extremely important in the examination, as there are often marks for uncovering the patient's 'hidden agenda'. Being an examination, and hence by definition an artificial situation, you will find the actor's healthcare-seeking motivation tends to be rather more neatly constructed than in clinical practice. For example, the patient experiencing vertigo may have underlying concerns of a brain tumour, which they will reveal with some gentle, empathetic questioning. Uncovering the patients' ICE – ideas (as to aetiology), concerns (hidden agendas) and expectations (as to treatment and prognosis) – is a useful framework for establishing this vital narrative information.

Chapter 1 details a number of common ENT presentations and the best method for tackling them in the examination or in clinical practice. We have detailed a number of specific areas that will need to be explored in the consultations, but it is important in each case that you start with general open questions. This will also help to establish a rapport with the patient, facilitating more specific questioning. Do remember that rapport, fluency and professionalism carry a lot of marks in the examination. Time is limited, of course, and it is also important to focus on the core symptoms and not be too distracted by interesting but fruitless diversions.

Joseph Manjaly and Peter Kullar

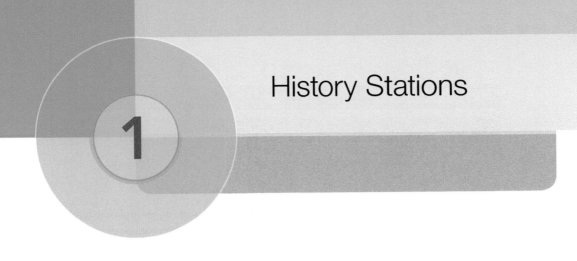

History Stations

There is always a history station in the examination. This chapter focuses on common presentations in the examination and ultimately reflects common scenarios in clinical practice. Each scenario starts with a short introduction. In the examination, there will be a similar introduction to read before you start the station. There is no allotted reading time, so read quickly but carefully.

For the history stations in the examination, you will only be expected to take a history – there is no requirement to examine the patient or to plan investigations. We have included a further discussion on investigations at the end of each section for reference.

DOI: 10.1201/b23029-1

RHINOLOGY

1.1   OLFACTORY DYSFUNCTION

A 70-year-old woman comes to your clinic reporting a change in her sense of smell for the last 2 months. Take a history from this patient.

Olfactory dysfunction (OD) has a potentially large number of causes and may have a significant impact on the patient's quality of life. Often it is the compromise of taste that the patient first notices.

OD can also lead to potentially dangerous situations, as the patient is unable to detect environmental hazards such as spoilt food or gas leaks. It is estimated that OD will affect 1% of the population under the age of 65 years and over 50% of the population older than 65 years.

GENERAL STRUCTURE OF THE CONSULTATION

An understanding of the olfactory pathway will be your basis for structuring the consultation, as a problem at any level of the pathway can cause OD.

The olfactory pathway starts with sensory neurons in the nose. These detect odorants and transmit via the olfactory nerve (cranial nerve I) to the olfactory bulb located on top of the cribriform plate at the base of the frontal lobe. These subsequently transmit to the olfactory cortex. There is also an ancillary pathway transmitting somatosensory information such as temperature via the trigeminal nerve (cranial nerve V).

Some useful terms to begin with are as follows:

- *Anosmia* – Absence of smell function
- *Hyposmia* – Decreased sensitivity to odorants
- *Hyperosmia* – Increased sensitivity to odorants
- *Cacosmia* – Sensation of foul smells
- *Phantosmia* – Olfactory hallucination

Structure your thinking around the possible causes of the OD. If you can work logically through these causes, you will not miss anything.

The OD can be

- *Conductive* – Anything that stops odorant molecules getting to the receptors in the nose
- *Sensory* – Loss of receptor function
- *Neural* – Damage of peripheral and central olfactory pathways

The most common causes of anosmia/hyposmia you will be expected to know are

- Sinonasal disease
- Post-viral anosmia (rhinovirus, coronavirus including COVID-19, parainfluenza virus)
- Head trauma
- Other, rarer causes (intracranial neoplasia; Turner's, Cushing's or Kallmann's syndrome)

SPECIFIC QUESTIONS

Start with an open question such as: 'I understand you are having some problems with your sense of smell. Perhaps you can tell me about this and how it's affecting you?'

This is a useful opening question, as it contextualises the patient's symptoms.

- When did you last have a normal sense of smell?
- Is it getting better or getting worse, or do you have bad episodes?
- Has there been any change since it started? Does your sense of smell fluctuate?
- Can you smell anything at all? Any unusual smells? (With this question you must be mindful that olfactory/auditory hallucinations can be a presenting feature of epilepsy. Patients often have preserved smell for noxious chemicals [e.g. strong perfume] through the trigeminal nerve.)
- Have you had any recent coughs or colds? (Post-viral OD is the most common aetiology, ask specifically about COVID-19.)
- Have you had any trauma to your head? (Trauma to the skull base can disrupt olfactory neurons passing through the cribriform plate.)
- Do you have any problems with your nose normally? (Particularly, ask about nasal obstruction, discharge and its quality, epistaxis, allergies and polyps. Ascertain whether symptoms are uni- or bilateral.)
- Have you had headaches, fits, faints, loss of consciousness or vomiting? (These are signs of raised intracranial pressure [ICP] and need to be asked about to rule out intracranial neoplasia, a rare but important cause of OD.)
- Have you noticed anything else? (Use this opportunity to screen for associated features of nasal disease such as swellings in the head and neck, paraesthesia, facial pain – remember pain, epistaxis, obstruction and paraesthesia are 'red flag' symptoms that may suggest a malignant cause for the OD.)
- Have you had any surgery on the nose? (Patients with ongoing sinonasal disease will often have had operative procedures. This correlates with OD as both cause and effect.)
- Have you noticed any change in your sense of taste? Does this interfere with eating?

PAST MEDICAL HISTORY AND GENERAL SYSTEMS REVIEW

- Do you have any medical problems? (Ask particularly about fevers, malaise, weight loss and systemic disease such as thyroid problems, diabetes and neurological conditions.)
- Have you noticed any changes in your memory? (Alzheimer's dementia and other neurodegenerative diseases have been associated with OD.)
- Do you have any children? (Explain that this may seem a strange question but Kallmann's syndrome [hypogonadotropic hypogonadism] can present with anosmia and impaired fertility.)

Close this part of the history by asking if the patient has anything else to add. This can be a useful time to screen for the patient's ideas, concerns and expectations.

DRUG HISTORY

- Are you taking any regular medication? (Ask particularly about antihypertensive and antihyperlipidaemic drugs, as these are known to be associated with OD.)
- Do you have any allergies to medications?

FAMILY HISTORY

- Do any conditions run in your family? (Ask about nasal polyposis, allergic rhinitis and cystic fibrosis, which predispose to conductive OD.)

SOCIAL HISTORY

- What do you do for work? (Try to discover if there has been any exposure to toxic chemicals, e.g. nickel.)
- Do you smoke cigarettes?
- Do you have any pets or exposure to animals? (Allergic rhinitis can lead to OD.)

FURTHER DISCUSSION: EXPLANATION AND PLANNING

Explain you would fully examine the patient's head and neck, obviously paying particular attention to the nose. Examine the nose in the standard fashion (see Chapter 2) paying attention to the nasal mucosa for signs of inflammation, deviation of the nasal septum and the presence of polyps. Explain you would perform nasal endoscopy with either the rigid or the flexible nasendoscope.

Explain that routinely other tests are only ordered as appropriate from the patient's history and examination findings and often no further investigation is helpful.

Blood tests can be used to rule out systemic disease (e.g. blood sugar, thyroid function tests).

If nasal pathology is detected on nasendoscopy (e.g. mucopus seen at the meatal orifices) and there are other features of chronic rhinosinusitis then a computed tomography (CT) of the paranasal sinuses can be ordered to delineate the degree of sinonasal disease, in planning for possible operative intervention.

CT imaging is also required if the patient presents with a constellation of 'red flag' symptoms as discussed.

If no nasal pathology is detected, then magnetic resonance imaging (MRI) of the head/olfactory pathway can be used to rule out uncommon tumours such as meningiomas and tumours of the olfactory cleft.

Further evaluation of smell can be performed using the University of Pennsylvania Smell Identification Test or Sniffin' Sticks (rarely used in clinical practice).

Discuss treatment options depending on results of the investigations (e.g. sinonasal disease, tumours).

If sensorineural anosmia (most often of post-viral origin) is diagnosed, explain that there are no curative treatments. Spontaneous recovery is possible, COVID-19 related anosmia typically improves in 7–14 days. In patients without spontaneous improvement there is some evidence that smell training (actively and mindfully sniffing four distinct scents daily) or vitamin A drops are helpful in some patients.

Patient reassurance and education are important, warning specifically about the risk of gas leaks and contaminated food.

1.2   NOSEBLEEDS IN ADULTS

A 45-year-old man attends your outpatient clinic reporting repeated nosebleeds over the last few months.

Although epistaxis is a common occurrence in all age groups, typically it has a bimodal distribution presenting in children and the elderly. The nose has a rich blood supply from both the internal (anterior and posterior ethmoid arteries) and external carotid arteries (facial and internal maxillary arteries). Bleeding is classically described as originating from the anterior or posterior septum, although the distinction between these is somewhat arbitrary. Anterior bleeds are most often from Kiesselbach plexus/Little's area, whereas posterior bleeds are more often from the sphenopalatine artery or are of venous origin.

GENERAL STRUCTURE OF THE CONSULTATION

Most cases will not have a singular cause but will be the result of a number of factors such as nasal trauma, rhinitis, hypertension and anticoagulation. These risk factors tend to increase with age, and hence the increasing prevalence in the elderly population. It is important to differentiate these cases from those that may have a more sinister cause, such as intranasal malignancy.

SPECIFIC QUESTIONS

- How long have you been having nosebleeds?
- How often do they occur?
- When you have a nosebleed, how long does it last?
- How much blood do you lose? (Measures such as an egg cup, teaspoon, etc. can be useful to quantify amounts.)
- Does it come from one side or both sides?
- Does blood come into the mouth? (This may be indicative of posterior bleeds.)
- What do you do to stop the bleeding? (This question can also ascertain whether the patient has an understanding of first aid.)
- Have you required hospital treatment to stop the bleeding in the past?
- Do you have any associated nasal symptoms? (Ask particularly about nasal obstruction, pain, discharge, crusting, paraesthesia and lymphadenopathy in the neck. These are 'red flag' symptoms for intranasal malignancy.)
- Have you had any trauma to the nose? (Particularly ask about nasal picking/scratching.)
- Are you exposed to animals/pollen? (Allergens are a common cause of epistaxis, by causing inflammation and hyperaemia of the nasal mucosa.)
- Ask about how the condition is affecting the patient, e.g. interfering with socialising.

PAST MEDICAL HISTORY AND GENERAL SYSTEMS REVIEW

- Ask about hypertension, heart disease, bleeding diatheses and liver disease.

These are all known bleeding risk factors.

DRUG HISTORY

- Do you take any blood-thinning tablets? (Particularly, warfarin, aspirin and clopidogrel.)
- Do you use intranasal oxygen? (This predisposes to epistaxis by drying the nasal mucosa.)
- Ask sensitively about intranasal drug use, e.g. cocaine.
- Do you have any allergies to medications?

FAMILY HISTORY

- Do any blood clotting disorders run in your family? (Hereditary coagulopathies predispose to epistaxis.)

SOCIAL HISTORY

- Do you smoke or drink alcohol? Smoking increases the risk of nasal squamous cell carcinoma (SCC).
- What is your occupation?

Occupational exposure to wood dust/flour/heavy metals is a risk factor for sinonasal malignancy.

FURTHER DISCUSSION: EXPLANATION AND PLANNING

Explain you would examine the patient's head and neck, paying particular attention to the nose and nasal septum.

Often with anterior bleeding points you can visualise a septal vessel that can be cauterised. A week of intranasal antibiotic such as Naseptin cream can then be prescribed.

If there is no obvious bleeding point to visualise on anterior rhinoscopy, you would perform rigid endoscopy.

Blood tests are rarely necessary. However, in cases of severe blood loss with suspected anaemia, or in cases where there is the suspicion of an underlying coagulopathy, a full blood count (FBC) and clotting profile should be ordered.

With patients on warfarin, the international normalised ratio (INR) should be checked (their 'yellow book' should document the normal range for their INR).

Patients with 'red flag' symptoms for neoplasia should undergo CT examination of the head, paranasal sinuses and neck.

If the patient does not have a working knowledge of first aid measures, then these should be explained. For example, place the head forwards and pinch the soft part of the nose, and ice on the back of the neck can also be tried.

Explain to the patient that any bleeds that do not stop with first aid require them to come in to hospital. Initially it is very likely that nasal cautery will be attempted; severe bleeding may require recourse to nasal packing and a stay as an inpatient.

In recurrent nosebleeds, refractory to more conservative management, surgical ligation of the bleeding vessel, e.g. sphenopalatine artery ligation or radiological embolisation, may be indicated.

1.3   NASAL CRUSTING

A 42-year-old woman attends the ear, nose and throat (ENT) clinic with a history of 'always having loads of stuff up my nose'.

GENERAL STRUCTURE OF THE CONSULTATION

This is a common presentation in ENT clinics and in the general population. In the majority of cases it requires no specific treatment. However, there are systemic conditions that can present with nasal crusting, so a thorough history is required. A chronic presentation without systemic symptoms is very likely to have a local cause such as atrophic rhinitis, trauma or rhinosinusitis.

SPECIFIC QUESTIONS

- What exact problems are you having with your nose? (It is important to ask open questions initially, particularly when the presenting complaint is quite vague.)
- How long have you been having problems?
- Do you have any other problems with the nose? (It is important to ask about nasal obstruction, which can be associated with polyps.)
- Do you have nasal whistling or changes in the 'gristle' of the nose? (This may indicate a septal perforation with overlying crust.)
- Do you have nosebleeds, facial weakness, sensory changes, changes in vision, facial pain or headaches? (These may be suggestive of underlying sinonasal malignancy.)
- Do you have any disturbance in your sense of smell? (Olfactory dysfunction – cacosmia may be indicative of atrophic rhinitis.)
- Ask about nasal picking. (This is the leading cause of septal perforation.)
- Have you had any other nasal trauma? (This includes nasogastric tube insertions and irradiation.)
- Do you have any problems with your ears? (An associated otitis media with effusion [OME] may be a sign of a nasopharyngeal malignancy but it may also indicate vasculitis (granulomatosis with polyangiitis [GPA]/eosinophilic GPA [EGPA]).
- Do you have any hearing loss? (GPA can cause a sensorineural hearing loss [SNHL] or mixed hearing loss.)

PAST MEDICAL HISTORY AND GENERAL SYSTEMS REVIEW

- Do you have any other medical conditions? (A full systems review is required in all cases as vasculitis and granulomatosis disease that can present with nasal crusting have manifestations in all areas of the body. Ask specifically about haematuria, haemoptysis, shortness of breath, paraesthesia, weaknesses and changes in vision.)
- Have you had any previous operations on the nose? (Particularly, septoplasty/septorhinoplasty.)

DRUG HISTORY

- Are you on any medications? (Include intranasal cocaine, as this can cause widespread nasal damage because of its vasoconstrictive properties as well as impurities in the preparations, as can home oxygen use through drying of the nasal mucosa and repeated trauma from nasal prongs.)
- Do you have any allergies to medications?

FAMILY HISTORY

- Do any conditions run in the family?

SOCIAL HISTORY

- Ask about travel history and ethnic heritage. (TB, acquired immune deficiency syndrome, syphilis, rhinoscleroma and leprosy are possible causes and the relevant investigations should be performed in at-risk individuals.)
- What do you do for work? (Ask about exposure to chrome salts. Workers in leather and nickel industries are particularly at risk. Woodworkers are at risk from sinonasal malignancy [most frequently, adenocarcinoma].)

FURTHER DISCUSSION: EXPLANATION AND PLANNING

A full examination of the nose should be undertaken using anterior rhinoscopy and rigid endoscopy. The areas of nasal crusting should be noted. The septum should be examined for perforations. Any suspicious areas should be biopsied (particularly, irregular or granulating mucosa).

Examine for fetor and polyps.

Granulomatous disease such as GPA causes irregular 'cobblestone' oedematous mucosa. EGPA predisposes to polyps and allergic rhinitis.

Plan a full examination of the ears including pure-tone audiometry (PTA)/tympanometry if indicated.

Treatment depends on the cause – in post-traumatic cases it is very likely that no treatment is appropriate.

If systemic features are detected in the history, a range of investigations may be appropriate. These include c-ANCA (cytoplasmic antineutrophil cytoplasmic antibodies)/p-ANCA (perinuclear antineutrophil cytoplasmic antibodies; investigating GPA/EGPA), angiotensin-converting enzyme (ACE) levels (investigating chest X-ray [CXR; investigating GPA) and FBC/urea and electrolytes (U+Es). (Anaemia is associated with sarcoidosis and eosinophilia is associated with EGPA.)

Plan a nasal septal biopsy if neoplasia is suspected.

Plan referral to other specialities where systemic disease is suspected, e.g. GPA patients are usually managed under the joint care of respiratory, renal and ENT physicians.

Further treatment includes nasal irrigation and humidification.

Surgical treatment involves repair of septal perforation. Radical procedures (e.g. Young's) are less popular.

1.4   CATARRH, POST-NASAL DRIP AND CHRONIC RHINOSINUSITS

A 47-year-old female shop worker reports the feeling of mucus running down the back of her throat. She tells you that her throat has been itchy for many years.

Catarrh is a non-specific term used by patients for a number of different symptom patterns. These range from a productive cough to nasal obstruction. The wide variety of symptoms requires careful history taking, as the causative factors are wide ranging. Typically, catarrh is defined as inflammation of the mucous membranes of the upper airways causing an excess of mucus. Patients often describe a feeling of mucus 'running down' their throat. In some patients, catarrh persists due to underlying organic disease such as allergies or abnormalities like nasal polyps. However, it is common that no underlying abnormality can be detected; where this is the case, education and reassurance are the mainstay of treatment.

GENERAL STRUCTURE OF THE CONSULTATION

This is often a difficult consultation and a bit of manoeuvring is required to align the patient's demands with what you can deliver as a clinician. It is important to differentiate patients who are actually overproducing mucus from those who only have the sensation that they are. It can be helpful to ask the patient to rank his or her symptoms in order of severity. It is common that patients present with a number of different chronic symptoms that they attribute to mucus overproduction, e.g. nausea, headaches and tiredness.

SPECIFIC QUESTIONS

- Ask the patient to describe the symptoms he or she is experiencing.
- How long have you had these symptoms?
- Are you getting better or worse?
- Do you get worse at a particular time?
- Do you have a cough?
- Is there any production of mucus with the cough? (Ask about the quality of the mucus – its colour, its consistency and the presence of blood. Many patients feel an inability to shift mucus from their chests [failed expectoration] and this can be a source of great anxiety and annoyance.)
- Do you have a blocked nose?
- Do you have any nasal discharge, sinus pain or anosmia? These may indicate underlying chronic rhinosinusitis (CRS), which can be defined as per the European Position Paper of Rhinosinusitis and Nasal Polyps 2020 (EPOS 2020) as:
  - Inflammation of the nose and paranasal sinuses with two or more symptoms, one of which should be nasal congestion or rhinorrhea/post-nasal drip
  - +/– reduced sense of smell or facial pain
  - And either: Endoscopic signs of nasal polyps and/or oedema of the middle meatus and/or mucopurulent discharge from the middle meatus
  - And/or CT evidence of sinus disease
  - Symptoms should be present for more than 3 months

- Do you have any allergies? (Sneezing fits and epiphora are symptoms of allergic rhinitis.)
- Do you have any facial pain? (The presence of pain may indicate underlying infection or sinusitis.)
- Screen for the patient's ideas, concerns and expectations.

PAST MEDICAL HISTORY AND GENERAL SYSTEMS REVIEW

- Ask about weight loss, malaise and fevers.
- Ask about any other systemic disease that can predispose to immune compromise and subsequent infection, e.g. diabetes, human immunodeficiency virus (HIV).

DRUG HISTORY

- Are you on any medications?
- Do you have any allergies to medications?

FAMILY HISTORY

- Do any conditions run in the family?

SOCIAL HISTORY

- Do you smoke or drink alcohol?
- What do you do for work?

FURTHER DISCUSSION: EXPLANATION AND PLANNING

Explain that you will examine the nose and post-nasal space (PNS) with anterior rhinoscopy and flexible nasendoscopy (FNE)/rigid endoscopy.

Plan treatment of chronic rhinosinusitis or allergies as appropriate. The management of CRS involves the use of intranasal steroids, saline douching, antibiotics (for immunomodulatory effect), courses of oral steroids and in appropriate patients the use of novel biologics (monoclonal antibody treatments). Where symptoms are failing to be controlled with medical therapy surgery will be considered.

If no organic cause for the nasal symptoms is found, reassurance and learning to cope with symptoms is the key management strategy. Investigations should not be used to reassure patients.

Nasal steroids may be of benefit in patients with post-nasal drip. Patients often find saline nasal rinses useful. Sipping ice cold water may help to break the cycle of throat clearing.

1.5 SEPTAL PERFORATION

A 62-year-old man has been referred to your clinic with nasal crusting and a sense of nasal obstruction for a number of years.

The nasal septum is the division between the left and right nostrils. It is composed of five structures: perpendicular plate of the ethmoid, vomer, cartilage, maxillary crest and palatine crest.

Perforations can be in either the anterior or the posterior part of the septum. They can be asymptomatic or they can cause a number of symptoms – particularly bleeding, nasal obstruction and nasal whistling.

GENERAL STRUCTURE OF THE CONSULTATION

As always, the structure of the consultation will follow possible causes of the disease. The most common causes are as follows:

- Traumatic causes (e.g. nose picking, external trauma)
- Iatrogenic causes (previous surgery, nasal cautery)
- Inflammatory causes (e.g. sarcoid, GPA)
- Infective causes (e.g. syphilis, tuberculosis [TB])
- Neoplastic causes (SCC, basal cell carcinoma, T-cell lymphoma)
- Other causes (chromium workers, illicit drugs such as cocaine)

SPECIFIC QUESTIONS

- What symptoms are you getting from your nose? (Many perforations are asymptomatic and it is not unusual to diagnose them incidentally when examining the nose for other reasons. Ask specifically about epistaxis, whistling, crusting and sense of nasal obstruction. These are most common with anterior perforations. Posterior perforations are often asymptomatic.)
- Do you generally have problems with your nose? (Ask specifically about sinusitis, discharge, infections and pain.)
- Have you had any recent trauma to the nose? (This should include nasal picking and excessively forceful sneezing or blowing of the nose.)
- Have you had any operations on the nose? (Perforations can arise as a complication of septoplasty and septorhinoplasty.)
- Have you had recurrent ear infections, sinusitis or chest infections? (This may prompt investigation for GPA.)
- Do you get any problems with your eyes? (Episcleritis and septal pathology may indicate autoimmune disease.)
- Explore the patient's ideas, concerns and expectations.

PAST MEDICAL HISTORY AND GENERAL SYSTEMS REVIEW

- Do you have any other medical conditions? (Ask specifically about autoimmune conditions and weight loss, fevers, lethargy and malaise [with neoplasia and granulomatous disease].)

DRUG HISTORY

- Are you on any medications? (Include use of intranasal illicit drugs such as cocaine.)
- Do you have any allergies to medications?

FAMILY HISTORY

- Do any conditions run in the family? (Ask specifically about autoimmune conditions.)

SOCIAL HISTORY

- Do you smoke or drink alcohol?
- What do you do for work? (Ascertain whether there has been exposure to noxious substances such as chrome or arsenic.)

FURTHER DISCUSSION: EXPLANATION AND PLANNING

Explain you would perform a full examination of the head and neck, focusing on the nose. Anterior rhinoscopy and rigid endoscopy can be used to delineate limits of perforation and to examine the PNS.

Unless there is an obvious cause, e.g. previous septal surgery, all patients should have baseline blood tests. These include FBC, U+Es (to check renal function, as systemic lupus erythematosus can cause renal failure) and erythrocyte sedimentation rate (ESR)/c-ANCA to assess for autoimmune conditions including GPA, ACE assay for sarcoidosis and Venereal Disease Research Laboratory (VDRL) test for syphilis.

Other tests include urine dipstick for microscopic haematuria with renal disease, CXR to rule out TB and sarcoidosis and biopsy, if there is a prominent granular area, to rule out neoplasia.

It is common that investigations do not reveal a cause.

Patients can be reassured that small septal perforations do not require any additional treatment.

For symptomatic perforations, nasal douching can be used to reduce crusting. If the patient is very troubled by symptoms, then consider for surgical repair.

Surgical options include a septal button for small anterior perforations. Surgical closure with a number of different flaps has been tried, including with a sliding mucoperichondrial, tunnelled buccal flap and anterior ethmoid artery flap. All of these operations have variable rates of success and there is very likely a large inter-surgeon variability in outcomes.

Patients diagnosed with autoimmune or granulomatous disease should be managed in conjunction with immunologist, renal or chest physicians.

1.6   NASAL OBSTRUCTION

A 54-year-old man presents with unilateral nasal obstruction and discharge affected the right side of his nose.

GENERAL STRUCTURE OF THE CONSULTATION

As always, the structure of the consultation will follow possible causes of the disease. The most common causes are as follows:

- Traumatic causes (e.g. external trauma and septal deviation)
- Iatrogenic causes (rhinitis medicamentosa)
- Inflammatory causes (e.g. allergy, autoimmune diseases)
- Infective causes (e.g. chronic rhinosinusitis)
- Neoplastic causes (e.g. polyps, sinonasal malignancy)
- Other causes

SPECIFIC QUESTIONS

- When was the onset of symptoms and the duration, including any history of trauma, upper respiratory tract infections (URTIs) or flu-like illness?
- Is the obstruction affecting one side or both?
- The persistence of symptoms is important to establish. Is the nose always blocked or does this come and go?
- A mechanical obstruction due to septal deviation will be persistent and typically unilateral. Fluctuating unilateral nasal obstruction, involving either side at any one time can relate to mucosal disease or the non-dominant nasal airway during the normal physiological nasal cycle.
- Are there any associated symptoms such as nasal discharge, post-nasal drip, change in smell sense (hyposmia/anosmia), itching, sneezing, epistaxis, facial pressure or pain and crusting? The nature, duration and severity of any associated symptoms should be established.
- Exacerbating factors may relate to seasonal or occupational exposures. Are symptoms worse any particular time of year, for example? This may suggest an allergic or irritant component to mucosal disease.
- Are there any known allergens/hayfever, e.g. grass, pollen, cats, dogs, dust mites?
- Are there red flags for sinonasal malignancy? (Red flags include unilateral symptoms, epistaxis, cacosmia, facial pain/paraesthesia, orbital symptoms and new neck lumps.)

PAST MEDICAL HISTORY AND GENERAL SYSTEMS REVIEW

- Is there any history of nasal polyposis, asthma, aspirin intolerance (Samter's triad), cystic fibrosis, coeliac disease or immunodeficiency?
- Has there been previous sinus or nasal surgery?

DRUG HISTORY

- Are you taking any regular medications? Include intranasal over-the-counter, prescription and recreational drug use. Persistent oxymetazoline (Otrivine) use can result in rhinitis medicamentosa.
- Do you have any allergies to medication?

FAMILY HISTORY

- Is there any history of nasal polyps, sinus disease, autoimmune disease or sinonasal malignancy in the family?

SOCIAL HISTORY

- Do you smoke or drink alcohol?
- What is your current and what was your previous occupation/exposures? (Ask specifically about nickel, chromium and wood chip dust.)

FURTHER DISCUSSION: EXPLANATION AND PLANNING

Explain that you would perform a thorough ENT examination including examination of the nose (anterior rhinoscopy), oropharynx, head and neck plus flexible nasendoscopy.

Additional tests may include nasal mist test, peak inspiratory flow rate and skin prick tests for common allergens.

The examination aims to establish the contribution of mucosal disease, structural abnormality or any intranasal lesion to symptoms. Further investigation will depend on findings and clinical suspicion but may include imaging (CT or MRI) and biopsy.

1.7   FACIAL PAIN

A 40-year-old female presents with a 2-year history of facial pain. There is pain in the cheeks and behind the eyes. A course of intranasal steroids and antibiotics has not improved her 'sinusitis' symptoms.

GENERAL STRUCTURE OF THE CONSULTATION

Facial pain is a common presentation in ENT clinics and in the general population. The structure of the consultation will follow possible causes of the disease, but it must be stressed that the medical history is critical in the diagnosis as the majority of patients will be normal on examination. The face has multiple innervations and referred pain must be considered. Broadly, facial pain can be divided into sinogenic and non-sinogenic in origin. Sinogenic facial pain can be caused due to acute chronic rhinosinusitis but is uncommon in chronic rhinosinusitis (CRS). Non-sinogenic facial pain has a number of causes, including neuropathic (e.g. migraine, tension headache, midfacial segment pain), cranial neuropathies (e.g. trigeminal neuralgia, trigeminal autonomic cephalgias), dental pain, temporomandibular pain and myofascial pain.

SPECIFIC QUESTIONS

- Tell me about the pain – Is it sharp or dull? Is it present on both sides of the face?
- When do you get the pain, is it there all the time?
- How does the pain affect your life?
- Any lethargy/headaches/aura/sensitivity to lights/sounds?
- Any autonomic features (tearing/nausea/vomiting)?
- Any symptoms of rhinosinusitis – Nasal blockage, rhinorrhoea, change/decrease in sense of smell?
- Anything that makes the symptoms worse? Ask about stress, caffeine intake.

PAST MEDICAL HISTORY AND GENERAL SYSTEMS REVIEW

- Ask about weight loss, malaise and fevers.
- Ask about migraine.
- Ask about recurrent headaches.
- Ask about dental and jaw problems.

FAMILY HISTORY

- Ask about migraine.

DRUG HISTORY

- Are you taking any regular medications? (Include intranasal steroids, analgesia and decongestants.)
- Do you have any allergies to medication?

SOCIAL HISTORY

- Do you smoke?

FURTHER DISCUSSION: EXPLANATION AND PLANNING

Explain that you would perform a thorough ENT examination, including examination of the nose (anterior rhinoscopy), oropharynx, head and neck plus flexible nasendoscopy, looking for signs of sino-nasal disease such as infection, oedema, inflammation, trauma and tumours.

Without the history or examination findings consistent with CRS, chronic facial pain alone is unlikely to be due to CRS and other causes should be ruled out. The examination should also include testing the cranial nerves, palpation for points of tenderness and trigger points, jaw clicks and dental pain.

Routine CT scan of the sinuses is discouraged as a diagnostic tool. MRI may be considered to look for intracranial pathology, or microvascular compromising of cranial nerve roots (trigeminal neuralgia).

Formal and long-term management of conditions that can be confused for sinusitis can be under the GP, neurology or dentists, however some basic features and management strategies for common conditions should be known.

Migraines are typically characterized by severe, asymmetrical, throbbing pain, with systemic symptoms such as nausea, lethargy, photophobia or phonophobia, and can last 4–72 hours sometimes with a preceding aura. They are most common in young women and approximately 70% of patients have a close family history of migraines. Management strategies include prophylactic medication (propranolol or topiramate) or symptomatic relief during migraine attacks (triptans and basic analgesia).

Tension-type headaches cause symmetrical dull pain in frontal, bitemporal or occipital regions and are non-debilitating unlike migraines. Midfacial segment pain is similar, but the pain is felt in the retro-orbital region, cheeks or nasion, with a pressure sensation but no airway obstruction and is commonly incorrectly attributed to sinonasal disease. The treatment for both conditions is primarily performed with amitriptyline.

Trigeminal neuralgia causes severe, sharp shooting pain in the distribution of the maxillary or mandibular divisions of the trigeminal nerve. It is typically unilateral and short lived but recurrent and can be induced by factors such as light touch, eating or exposure to cold air. They may have autonomic features such as lacrimation, conjunctival injection, nasal congestion, rhinorrhoea, ptosis or diaphoresis. Treatment is performed with the anticonvulsant medication carbamazepine.

PAEDIATRICS

1.8   SNORING IN A CHILD

A mother attends with her 5-year-old boy and is worried that he is snoring loudly and sometimes stops breathing at night.

GENERAL STRUCTURE OF THE CONSULTATION

Sleep-disordered breathing is common in the paediatric population and encompasses a spectrum from simple snoring to obstructive sleep apnoea (OSA). The history is important as it determines whether further investigations are required, and aids operative planning as to whether overnight monitoring or operating in a unit with a paediatric intensive care unit (PICU) is required. In this station you will be talking to an actor playing the parent. There will not be a child present.

SPECIFIC QUESTIONS

- Tell me about what happens at night.
- Does he breathe through his mouth?
- Does he ever stop breathing or hold his breath?
- Does he ever make sounds like he is choking in his sleep?
- Does he have symptoms of rhinitis?
- Does he suffer with tonsillitis?
- Does he wet the bed?
- Is he irritable when he wakes up? Does he demonstrate hyperactivity during the day? Is he sleepy during the day? (Daytime sleepiness is less prevalent in children and often they suffer with daytime hyperactivity instead.)
- Are there any behavioural problems?
- How is he performing at school? Does he suffer with poor concentration? Any concerns with hearing?

PAST MEDICAL HISTORY AND GENERAL SYSTEMS REVIEW

- Have there been any admissions to hospital?
- Has he had previous surgery?
- Are there any other medical problems or syndromes?
- What is his weight and height – Are there any signs of failure to thrive?

FAMILY HISTORY

- Ask about any conditions that run in the family.

DRUG HISTORY

- Is he on any medications?
- Does he have any allergies to medications?

SOCIAL HISTORY

- Does he have any siblings? If so, does the sibling have similar problems?

FURTHER DISCUSSION: EXPLANATION AND PLANNING

- Parents sometimes bring on their phones videos of their child sleeping which can be very useful in further assessing the severity of the symptoms.
- It is important to look for any signs of craniofacial syndromes as these may be undiagnosed and increase the risk of OSA.
- Obesity is increasing in the paediatric population and there are increased rates of OSA in this subgroup.
- In healthy children it is not usually necessary to perform a sleep study. If there are signs of obesity, craniofacial disproportion, small tonsils or neuromuscular disease then a sleep study should be performed.
- Consider where the most appropriate place to perform surgery will be – Do you require a PICU for this child? Children under 1, <10kg or with comorbidities e.g. cerebral palsy, Down syndrome, neuromuscular disorders should be operated on in centres with PICU support.

1.9   RECURRENT TONSILLITIS

A 10-year-old child presents to the outpatients clinic, accompanied by the child's parent, with a history of recurrent tonsillitis.

GENERAL STRUCTURE OF THE CONSULTATION

The palatine tonsils form part of Waldeyer's ring of lymphoid tissue in the pharynx along with the adenoid pad, lingual tonsils and mucosa-associated lymphoid tissue (MALT). They sit within the tonsillar fossa, bordered anteriorly by the palatoglossal arch (anterior pillar) and posteriorly by the palatopharyngeal arch (posterior pillar). Acute tonsillitis involves inflammation of the palatine tonsillar tissue and is extremely common, especially in the paediatric population; and contributes to missed days of school and work every year. There are other causes of 'sore throats' that are worth bearing in mind including viral upper respiratory tract infections, pharyngitis, and in the adult population, *Candida*, gastro-oesophageal reflux and malignancy.

The history is vital for both diagnosis and importantly establishing frequency of episodes and the impact on the child e.g. affect on schooling. In the exam setting it is important to remember the potential 'hidden agenda' that could be held by the parents, in this case arranging a tonsillectomy for their child. Acute tonsillitis can be viral or bacterial in origin, with group A beta-haemolytic streptococcus being the most common organism. Glandular fever, secondary to Epstein–Barr virus, can present similarly to acute bacterial tonsillitis, with a typically longer history of symptoms. There are other viral causes including adenovirus and respiratory syncytial virus which may be complicated by superadded bacterial infection.

SPECIFIC QUESTIONS

In this setting the history is mainly taken from the parent.

* What symptoms does the child have during the acute episodes and how bad are they?

A clue to this would be whether the child required antibiotics or hospital admission.

* How many episodes are they having and how much time has been missed from school?
* Is there previous history of peritonsillar abscess (quinsy), although uncommon in children?
* Is the child well between episodes/able to return to normal diet?
* Are there any new/persistent/growing lumps in the head and neck? (These are red flags for lymphoma in a child who is failing to thrive with recurrent episodes of tonsillitis and/or tonsillar asymmetry. Further enquiry into B-symptoms and family history should be sought.)
* Are there problems with snoring or apnoea? (This could suggest sequelae of enlarged obstructing palatine tonsils including obstructive sleep apnoea. A history of mouth breathing or recurrent otitis media effusion 'glue ear' with hearing loss may be suggestive of enlarged adenoid tissue.)

PAST MEDICAL HISTORY AND GENERAL SYSTEMS REVIEW

* Are there any other medical problems or syndromes?
* Any previous surgery?
* What is the child's weight and height – Are there any signs of failure to thrive?

FAMILY HISTORY

- Does the child have siblings with similar issues?
- Try to illicit the mother's ideas, concerns and expectations, as it is likely she may have a 'hidden agenda'.

DRUG HISTORY

- Are they on any regular medications?
- Do they have any allergies to medication?

SOCIAL HISTORY

- Does he have any siblings? If so, does the sibling have similar problems?

FURTHER DISCUSSION: EXPLANATION AND PLANNING

Explain that you would perform a thorough ENT examination including oropharynx (the tonsils' symmetry and size should be noted and graded using the Brodsky grading system (1–4), otoscopy for signs of glue ear, head and neck examination and mist test.

The indications for tonsillectomy include recurrent tonsillitis, tonsillar asymmetry for histological diagnosis, obstructive sleep apnoea and recurrent quinsy.

The Scottish Intercollegiate Guidelines Network (SIGN) guideline on management of sore throats and indications for tonsillectomy are well established and aid selection of best candidates for surgery, and can be referred to when counselling a patient or parent. This is equally useful to refer to when offering tonsillectomy and justifying why surgery is not indicated, in addition to quoting the established risks of this operation.

SIGN guidelines are as follows:

- Sore throats are due to acute tonsillitis.
- Episodes of sore throat are disabling and prevent normal function.
- Seven or more well-documented, clinically significant, adequately treated sore throats in the preceding year, five or more episodes in each of the preceding 2 years and three or more episodes in each of the preceding 3 years.

1.10   NOSEBLEEDS IN CHILDREN

A 10-year-old girl comes to clinic with her mother who tells you the child has been having two or three nosebleeds a week for the last year.

Nosebleeds are a common complaint in children. The vast majority are not serious; however, they are often a source of serious parental concern and a source of social embarrassment for the child. As with adult epistaxis, bleeds can be classified on their site of origin: either anterior or posterior. Anterior bleeds from the Little's area (where arteries from internal and external carotids anastomose) are the most common. In older children most epistaxis result from nasal trauma or nasal picking; however, nasal foreign bodies are also common.

GENERAL STRUCTURE OF THE CONSULTATION

This is a similar structure to the history for nosebleeds in adults (*see* Section 1.2), with some specific additions. You will be faced with an actor playing the parent; there will never be children in the examination. Think about the possible causes of a nosebleed in a child to help structure your approach to this station.

CAUSES INCLUDE

- Nasal picking
- Allergies
- Infection
- Trauma
- Very rarely, neoplasia

SPECIFIC QUESTIONS

- How long has she been having nosebleeds?
- How often do they occur?
- How long do they last?
- How much blood does she lose? (Refer to familiar quantities such as an egg cup to help the mother here.)
- Does it come from one side or from both sides?
- Does it come into the mouth?
- What do you do to stop the bleeding?
- Has she had any treatment in the past?
- Are there any associated nasal symptoms? (Ask particularly about nasal obstruction, pain, discharge, crusting, paraesthesias, and swellings in the head and neck. These are 'red flag' symptoms for intranasal malignancy.)
- Has she had any trauma to the nose? (Particularly ask about nasal picking.)
- What is the impact on her life? (Ask about problems at school – recurrent nosebleeds can be socially isolating.)
- Does she have any exposure to animals/pollen? (Allergens are a common cause of epistaxis, by causing inflammation and hyperaemia of the nasal mucosa.)
- Try to elicit the mother's ideas, concerns and expectations, as it is very likely she will be anxious about serious underlying pathology.

PAST MEDICAL HISTORY AND GENERAL SYSTEMS REVIEW

- Is she otherwise well? (Ask about weight and development, fevers and malaise. These are useful questions for ruling out systemic disease.)
- Has she had any unexpected bruising or bleeding from other sites? (Many haematological disorders can present with epistaxis, e.g. childhood leukaemias.)

DRUG HISTORY

- Is she on any medications?
- Does she have any allergies to medications?

FAMILY HISTORY

- Do any conditions run in the family?

SOCIAL HISTORY

- Does she have any siblings? If so, does the sibling have similar problems?
- Is there any smoking in the household? (This predisposes to epistaxis by irritating the nasal mucosa.)

FURTHER DISCUSSION: EXPLANATION AND PLANNING

Explain you would examine the child's head and neck, paying particular attention to the nose and nasal septum. The first line treatment would be a 10-day course of intranasal antibiotic cream such as Naseptin. Cautery is a second-line therapy, as it is often difficult in children. If you are unable to perform a satisfactory examination and the child is having severe symptoms, then an examination under anaesthetic may be appropriate.

Rigid endoscopy is surprisingly well tolerated by children and should be performed if there is no initially obvious cause for the bleeding.

Explain blood tests are not usually required but may be appropriate in heavy recurrent bleeds or when there is suspicion of an underlying haematological condition.

In exceptional cases, MRI of the head may be appropriate to rule out neoplasia.

Reassure appropriately, as most children will grow out of nosebleeds. Often a short course of Naseptin is all that is needed.

Educate the parent about first aid techniques if he or she is not familiar with them.

1.11   HEARING LOSS IN A CHILD

A 4-year-old girl comes to your clinic with her mother who is concerned about the child's hearing.

The Newborn Hearing Screening Programme was set up in the UK in 2005 and aims to identify children with a >40dB congenital hearing loss in the better ear. There are two screening pathways: well baby and NICU/SCBU pathway. Automated otoacoustic emissions (AOAEs) are used as the initial screening test. Those babies who fail the first test (which may or may not be due to an underlying hearing deficit) are retested with AOAEs and automated auditory brainstem responses.

For the purposes of the examination, the most likely scenario will be dealing with hearing loss in older children. The most common cause of hearing impairment in this patient population is OME. This common condition is most often self-limiting, and a period of 6 months' watchful waiting will result in 90% of children spontaneously recovering. However, this is not always the case, and the hearing impairment may compromise speech and language development.

GENERAL STRUCTURE OF THE CONSULTATION

The differential for hearing loss in a child is broad; however, this can be significantly narrowed through careful history taking and examination.

SPECIFIC QUESTIONS

- Has she had recurrent ear infections? (In approximately 50% of OME cases there has been a preceding acute otitis media [AOM], particularly in younger children.)
- Has she complained of earache? (Ask also about ear tugging, discharge, fevers, irritability, nausea and poor feeding as signs of AOM.)
- What have you noticed about her hearing? (Ask specifically about interaction with siblings and parents at home, her progress at school and whether she insists on an elevated television volume.)
- Does she snore or have any breathing problems? (Adenoidal hypertrophy may be associated with obstructive sleep apnoea and Eustachian tube dysfunction leading to OME).
- Has she had any recent trauma to the head? (Temporal bone fractures can result in auditory nerve compromise.)
- Are there any concerns about the development of her speech and language?
- It can be useful to compare development with siblings or peer group. This is a good point to explore the parent's ideas, concerns and expectations.

PAST MEDICAL HISTORY AND GENERAL SYSTEMS REVIEW

- Is she normally well in herself? (Ask about Down's syndrome, cleft palate and other developmental delay that is associated with OME.)
- Has she had her routine immunisations?

- Was she a full-term baby? (Ask about birth and perinatal history and prematurity, including maternal infections such as TORCH [toxoplasmosis, other, rubella, cytomegalovirus, herpes simplex virus] infections that have been linked to SNHL.)

DRUG HISTORY

- Is she on any medications?
- Any allergies to medications?

FAMILY HISTORY

- Do any conditions run in the family? (Family history of hearing loss/SNHL can have a genetic basis [both recessive and dominant].)

SOCIAL HISTORY

- Is there any smoking in the household? (This has been shown to be associated with OME in children.)

FURTHER DISCUSSION: EXPLANATION AND PLANNING

Explain you would perform full examination of both ears including otoscopy, tympanometry and age-appropriate hearing tests, including air and bone thresholds as appropriate.

Treatment – The most common cause of hearing loss in this population is OME. Treatment is in accordance with NICE guidelines. If there is history of hearing loss of 25–30 dB hearing loss and clinical evidence of bilateral OME then it is reasonable to initially consider a 3-month watchful waiting period. If symptoms are not improving and there is concomitant morbidity (e.g. failure to progress at school), then it may be appropriate to consider surgical management (myringotomy plus grommet insertion, with or without adenoidectomy).

Advice can be given about managing at home and school (e.g. minimising background noise, listening aids in the classroom and working with teaching assistants).

Hearing aids can also be considered.

Genetic screening may be appropriate in patients with SNHL. Plan referral to paediatrician if there is suspicion of a syndromic cause.

Unilateral hearing loss in children is usually managed with lifestyle measures or a hearing aid (air or bone conduction device).

Children with bilateral severe to profound SNHL may be considered for cochlear implantation. Current NICE guidelines recommend consideration of cochlear implantation for people with thresholds of an average of >80 dB in the better ear at two frequencies between 0.5 and 4 kHz who receive inadequate benefit from hearing aids. For children, adequate benefit is defined as speech, language and listening skills that are appropriate for age, cognitive and developmental stage. The NICE guidance for suitability of cochlear implantation is due to be updated in 2022.

1.12   CHILD WITH RECURRENT EAR INFECTIONS

A 4-year-old girl attends your ENT clinic with a history of recurrent 'ear infections'.

GENERAL STRUCTURE OF THE CONSULTATION

Here it is important to find out what type of infection the child is getting. In the examination setting there will never be a child at the station; instead, your questioning will be directed to the parent. AOM is the most common presentation in this age group. However, this needs to be differentiated from other infections (e.g. otitis externa [OE], although this is rare in childhood).

AOM is an inflammation of the middle ear manifesting with both local and systemic symptoms. Common symptoms include otalgia, discharge, fever, ear tugging, nausea and decreased appetite.

The causative agent is often viral (respiratory syncytial virus, adenovirus) but it can also be bacterial (*Streptococcus pneumoniae, Haemophilus influenzae*). There is increasing evidence that the microbiology of AOM is changing with the introduction of the polyvalent pneumococcal vaccine.

AOM is an extremely common condition, with almost all children having at least one episode. Approximately 10% of children experience four or more episodes in a year. AOM has a negative impact on the quality of life of both the child and the parents. It is important to remember AOM has potentially serious sequelae, including intracranial abscess and meningitis.

SPECIFIC QUESTIONS

- What symptoms is she getting? (Ask specifically about ear tugging, ear discharge, feeding patterns, fevers and lethargy.)
- How long has she been getting episodes?
- How frequent are the episodes?
- How long do the episodes last?
- Has she received antibiotics in the past?
- Has she been unwell recently? (Ask specifically about coughs, colds and rhinorrhea. AOM is often preceded by upper respiratory tract infections [URTIs]. Before 6 months there is passive immunity from transplacental IgG. In older children, recurrent cases may need investigation for immunocompromise, particularly if there are other recurrent infections, e.g. URTI.)
- How is her hearing and speech and language development? (It can be helpful to make a comparison with any other children in the family or the child's peer group at school.)
- How is she managing at school? Have the teachers noticed anything?
- Does the child snore at night? (Ask about signs of sleep apnoea or nasal obstruction that can predispose to AOM and OME.)

PAST MEDICAL HISTORY AND GENERAL SYSTEMS REVIEW

- Is she normally well in herself?
- Has she had her routine immunisations? (There is some evidence that the pneumococcal vaccine reduces the risk of AOM.)

- Has she had any other infections? (Any history of other infections may be suggestive of immunocompromise.)
- Was she a full-term baby? (Ask about the foetal and neonatal history.)

DRUG HISTORY

- Is she on any medications?
- Does she have any allergies to medications?

FAMILY HISTORY

- Do any conditions run in the family?

SOCIAL HISTORY

- Is there any smoking in the household? (This is an important environmental risk factor.)
- Are any siblings of the child affected similarly?

FURTHER DISCUSSION: EXPLANATION AND PLANNING

Explain you would perform a full examination of the child's head and neck, centring on the ears and the mouth (for cleft palate) and nose (for obstruction).

An irritable, clinically unwell child with the classic bulging, red tympanic membrane (TM) on otoscopy is diagnostic of AOM.

Often the TM has perforated and the canal is filled with pus. Middle ear pus can be distinguished from OE by its quality and pulsatility (due to middle ear vasculature).

Perform age-appropriate hearing tests.

The general body of evidence is that AOM should be treated with antibiotics in children <18 months old. In older children, a watchful waiting period of 48–72 hours is reasonable. Failure to progress after this time is indication for antibiotics (at the expense of increased risk of side effects).

Recurrent AOM can be treated with low-dose daily amoxicillin. As appropriate, it may be necessary to screen for immunocompromise with levels of serum immunoglobulins.

Myringotomy and grommet insertion is a reasonable treatment for children with recurrent disease, particularly if there are frequent infections with perforations and discharge.

HEAD AND NECK

1.13   NECK LUMP

A 58-year-old man attends the ENT clinic after noticing a lump in his neck.

GENERAL STRUCTURE OF THE CONSULTATION

Neck lumps are common both in examinations and in clinical practice. In children they are normally a benign reactive lymphadenopathy; in adults the majority are malignant. There are a number of potential causes and the likelihood of each depends on the patient demographic and the history.

COMMON CAUSES INCLUDE

- Congenital (seen in children and adults)
  - Branchial cyst
  - Thyroglossal cyst
  - Laryngocele
  - Teratoma
  - Dermoid cyst
  - Cystic hygroma
- Infective (seen in adults and children)
  - Viral lymphadenopathy
  - Bacterial lymphadenopathy
  - Granulomatous disease, e.g. sarcoid, TB
- Neoplastic (particularly in adults)
  - Metastatic SCC
  - Thyroid masses
  - Lymphoma
- Vascular (particularly in adults)
  - Carotid aneurysm
  - Carotid body tumour

SPECIFIC QUESTIONS

- When did you first notice the lump? (A short history, single, firm, lateral lump: often malignant or reactive. A short history, multiple, rubbery lumps: lymphoma, glandular fever, TB. A longer history, single and lateral lump: branchial cyst. A longer history, single, midline lump: thyroid mass, thyroglossal cyst.)
- Is it getting larger? (Malignant nodes tend to enlarge rapidly. Infective nodes often accompany a URTI.)
- Do you have any nasal blockage? (This can be associated with lesions in the PNS, e.g. nasopharyngeal carcinoma.)
- Do you have any pain in the ears? (Head and neck primaries often present with otalgia.)

- Do you have any pain in the throat? (This can be associated with head and neck primaries, and also with infective conditions such as glandular fever and tonsillitis.)
- Have you noticed any change in your voice? (Voice change and hoarseness are a 'red flag' for neoplasia.)
- Have you had any trouble swallowing? (Pharyngeal lesions may mechanically obstruct swallowing.)
- Do you smoke cigarettes?
- Do you drink alcohol? (Alcohol and smoking are risk factors for head and neck neoplasia.)
- Have you lost any weight? (Weight loss is associated with neoplasia [SCC, lymphoma] and infective conditions such as TB.)
- How is your appetite?
- Have you had any night sweats?
- Have you had any fevers? (Fevers and night sweats are associated with lymphoma and infective conditions such as TB.)
- Have you had any holidays abroad lately? (This is a risk factor for TB.)
- Have you had a recent chest infection or URTI? (A very common cause of reactive lymphadenopathy.)
- Does the lump change with eating? (Salivary masses often change with eating.)

PAST MEDICAL HISTORY AND GENERAL SYSTEMS REVIEW

- Do you have any other medical conditions? (Ask about general health including cardiovascular disease and diabetes.)
- Explore the patient's ideas, concerns and expectations.

DRUG HISTORY

- Are you on any medications?
- Do you have any allergies to medications?

FAMILY HISTORY

- Do any conditions run in the family?

SOCIAL HISTORY

- What do you do for work? (Check for exposure to chemicals and animals, e.g. abattoir work may increase susceptibility to rare infections such as brucellosis.)

FURTHER DISCUSSION: EXPLANATION AND PLANNING

Explain that you will perform a full ENT examination including fibreopotic nasendoscopy. This will include examination of the PNS, base of tongue, tonsils, pharynx, larynx and thyroid.

Examine the lump for size, site, character, pulsatility, mobility and transillumination. Perform ultrasound guided FNA (for microbiology/cytology).

Plan blood tests including FBC, white cell count, ESR and C-reactive protein. Special tests are infectious mononucleosis screen, HIV, CXR, barium swallow (with any dysphagia), MRI of the head and neck/CT chest (for staging if the lump is very likely to be neoplastic).

PET-CT/Panendoscopy and tonsillectomy/tongue based mucosectomy is indicated if there is a high index of suspicion for malignant disease/positive FNA and the original examination was unable to locate a primary.

The results of these investigations should be discussed at the head and neck MDT where a treatment plan will be decided.

1.14   DRY MOUTH

A 70-year-old man complains of a dry mouth for the last 6 months.

Saliva is produced from three pairs of major salivary glands (parotid, submandibular and sublingual) and multiple minor salivary glands throughout the mouth. Saliva is primarily water, with small quantities of dissolved mucus, enzymes and electrolytes. The main role of saliva is to aid the production of a moistened food bolus that can be swallowed. The presence of salivary enzymes amylase and lipase also plays an initial role in digestion. The normal adult produces and subsequently swallows approximately 1 L of saliva every day.

Salivation is under control of the autonomic nervous system. The decreased production of saliva is a normal physiological part of the 'fight-or-flight response' (sympathetic overdrive). However, a persistent dry mouth can become a source of morbidity, making chewing, eating and talking difficult.

GENERAL STRUCTURE OF THE CONSULTATION

The correct medical term for a dry mouth is xerostomia, defined as the real or apparent sensation of hyposalivation.

It is important to think about possible causes for the dry mouth to help structure your thinking when approaching this station. Disruption to any part of the pathway from the brain to the salivary gland can cause a reduction in the production of saliva.

You should consider sensory (disruption to taste sensation can cause hyposalivation), neural (damage to any part of the neural pathway, including cranial nerves VII, IX and V) and secretomotor dysfunction (direct damage to the salivary glands).

COMMON CAUSES INCLUDE

- Medication side effects – Any drug with effects on the autonomic nervous system can cause xerostomia e.g. antihypertensives and antidepressants.
- Mouth breathing – This may be due to nasal blockage, e.g. from adenoidal hypertrophy.
- Systemic disease – Autoimmune disease such as Sjögren's syndrome must be ruled out. Other systemic disease such as HIV, diabetes and Parkinson's disease can also cause dry mouth.
- Radiation therapy – The salivary glands, particularly the parotid glands, are often in the radiation field during treatment of head and neck cancer. A number of new developments including intensity-modulated radiotherapy have been developed to minimise collateral damage to healthy salivary tissue.
- Pseudoxerostomia – Rarely as a manifestation of psychiatric disease.

SPECIFIC QUESTIONS

- How long has your mouth been dry?
- Is it dry all the time or in episodes?
- Is it dry when you are eating? Does the sensation of dryness stop you eating?

- Do you have any problems with your senses of taste and smell?
- Do you have any problems swallowing? (Swallowing problems are a 'red flag' and should heighten your awareness of underlying malignancy.)
- Do you feel that you don't have enough saliva in your mouth?
- Do you sleep well? Do you snore? (Disturbed sleep and snoring predispose to loss of hydration of the oral mucosa.)
- Do you breathe through your nose or mouth? (Nasal obstruction can predispose to mouth breathing and hence dryness of the oral mucosa.)
- Do you have bad breath? Do you have any problems with your teeth or infections of the mouth? (The loss of saliva increases the growth of pathogenic oral microflora and hence the risk of cavities and intra-oral infection.)
- Screen for the patient's ideas, concerns and expectations.

PAST MEDICAL HISTORY AND GENERAL SYSTEMS REVIEW

- Are you usually well? (Ask specifically about diabetes, autoimmune disease and neurological disease.)
- Have you had any recent coughs or colds?
- Have you noticed any dryness of the eyes, rashes, arthritis or Raynaud's phenomenon? (These are the symptoms of Sjögren's syndrome.)
- Have you had any cancers of the head and neck region? (Ask specifically about radiation exposure.)

DRUG HISTORY

- Are you on any medications? (This is an extremely common cause of a dry mouth and a number of different classes of medication have xerostomia listed as a side effect.)
- Do you have any allergies to medications?

FAMILY HISTORY

- Does anyone in your family suffer from a similar problem? (Ask specifically about a history of autoimmune disease.)

SOCIAL HISTORY

- Do you smoke or drink alcohol?
- Ask sensitively about risk factors for HIV exposure (sexual history, intravenous drug use).
- What do you do for work? (Ask about voice abuse, e.g. teachers, singers – a rare but possible cause of a dry mouth.)

FURTHER DISCUSSION: EXPLANATION AND PLANNING

Explain you would examine the patient's head and neck fully, paying particular attention to the mouth and salivary glands.

Other investigations will depend on the history and examination findings. Blood glucose levels/HbA1C levels can be suggested if diabetes is suspected.

Plan FBC, U+Es, liver function tests, immunological tests including rheumatoid factor, ANA and SS-A, SS-B (Sjögren's syndrome A- and B-antibodies) if autoimmune disease is suspected. Sialometry can be used to quantify saliva production, but this is very rarely used outside of a research setting.

Plan biopsy of a minor salivary gland for histology to diagnose primary Sjögren's syndrome.

Plan imaging studies such as magnetic resonance sialography or more commonly ultrasound scan (USS) of the major salivary glands if primary salivary gland disease is suspected.

Treatment depends on the cause, e.g. stringent glucose control in diabetes, medication rationalisation, stopping smoking or referral to rheumatology service if an autoimmune condition is diagnosed.

Symptom management consists of frequent oral lubrication with fluids, artificial saliva, sialogogues (e.g. pilocarpine) and the use of chewing gum to stimulate saliva production.

1.15   LUMP IN THE THROAT

A 55-year-old lawyer presents to your outpatient clinic with a feeling of something in her throat for the last 4 months.

GENERAL STRUCTURE OF THE CONSULTATION

The feeling of something in the throat (FOSIT) has multiple potential causes. Generally, these can be split into benign and malignant. The majority of cases will be idiopathic (globus pharyngeus) in origin, with reassurance and education being the mainstay of treatment. It is crucial to rule out malignant disease. However, malignancy rarely presents solely with FOSIT. Therefore, the history is vital in diagnosis of the underlying problem. Another point to mention is that in the examination setting, these patients often have a 'hidden agenda' or specific worries about what might be causing their symptoms. There will be marks for finding out the cause of their anxiety.

SPECIFIC QUESTIONS

- Ask the patient to describe in her own words exactly the sensation she is getting. (Sensations range from a feeling of phlegm running down or sticking at the back of the throat to foreign body sensation with dysphagia.)
- How long have you had this sensation?
- Is it getting better or worse? (Globus pharyngeus is normally a non-progressive condition.)
- Does it come in episodes or is it present all the time?
- Is it better when eating? Has it ever interfered with eating? (Classically globus sensation goes away when swallowing, but this is not always the case.)
- Do you have any pain or trouble swallowing? (This is an important question, as any dysphagia or odynophagia should prompt further questioning and investigation. Important features include the time course, progression, worsening with solids or liquid [worse with liquids implies neurological disease] and regurgitation [pharyngeal pouch].)
- Have there been any changes in your voice? (Voice change is a 'red flag' symptom for upper aerodigestive tract neoplasia [*see* Section 1.16, 'Hoarse voice'].)
  - Do you clear your throat a lot?
- Do you have any new lumps in the head or neck? (Lymphadenopathy is an important feature of both infection and malignancy.)
- Do you suffer from heartburn or regurgitation?
- Do you have any pain in your ears? (Referred otalgia is a 'red flag' symptom for neoplasia of the head and neck [*see* Section 1.22].)

PAST MEDICAL HISTORY AND GENERAL SYSTEMS REVIEW

- Screen for weight loss, fevers, malaise, chest symptoms such as haemoptysis and shortness of breath.
- Ask about systemic illnesses and particularly screen for depression and psychiatric problems, including other healthcare-seeking behaviour or medically unexplained symptoms.

DRUG HISTORY

- Do you take any medications?
- Do you have any allergies to medications?

FAMILY HISTORY

- Do any conditions run in your family?

SOCIAL HISTORY

- Do you smoke or drink alcohol?
- What do you do for work?
- Ask about general anxiety levels and worries. It is important to try to explore the patient's ideas, concerns and expectations, as frequently these patients have a 'hidden agenda'.

FURTHER DISCUSSION: EXPLANATION AND PLANNING

Explain you would perform a thorough examination of the neck, including the neck lymph nodes and thyroid gland.

Explain you would perform flexible nasendoscopy to rule out any lesions of the upper aerodigestive tract.

If no abnormalities have been found and the history is suggestive of globus pharyngeus, then the patient can be reassured. Often a reassurance that there is no abnormality detected is all that the patient needs. In the clinical setting it can be useful to allow the patient to see his or her own aerodigestive tract using the flexible nasendoscope and video stack.

In patients who remain anxious, it is important for them to remove focus from the sensation. They should be encouraged to break the swallow-sensation cycle where dry swallowing/throat clearing worsens the sensation rather than eases it.

If the history and examination prove normal, further investigation such as barium swallows is generally not required. This is particularly true in younger non-smokers.

Laryngopharyngeal reflux (LPR) has been implicated in globus sensation; however, the efficacy of proton-pump inhibitors (PPIs) is still debated. Gaviscon Advance after meals and before bed time is helpful in reducing the effect of pepsin on the throat. The role of cognitive behavioural therapy (CBT) is also equivocal.

If more worrisome symptoms are revealed in the history, such as weight loss, constant and progressive dysphagia or pain (e.g. referred otalgia or odynophagia), then further investigation will be required. The first-line investigation is a barium swallow and/or rigid endoscopy with or without biopsies. Many head and neck surgeons will perform panendoscopy as a first-line treatment in any patient they feel is at high risk of malignancy.

1.16   HOARSE VOICE

A 64-year-old ex-publican presents to the outpatient clinic with a 4-month history of a hoarse voice.

The production of the human voice can be divided into three parts:

1. Production of airflow from the lungs
2. Vibration of the vocal folds
3. Articulation from the soft palate and tongue

A dysphonia is a disorder of the ability to produce normal vocal sounds and it can result from impairment at any part of the vocal tract.

GENERAL STRUCTURE OF THE CONSULTATION

This is a common presentation in outpatients and, as ever, there are a multiplicity of causes, both functional and organic. It is of the utmost importance to differentiate those of a benign from those of a malignant nature. The most common dysphonic voice is a hoarse voice. The most common reason for hoarseness is the interruption of normal vocal fold vibration.

The most common causes that you will be expected to know for the examination are

* Laryngitis – This can be either infective (viral/bacterial) or caused by local irritants such as smoking or LPR.
* Voice abuse – This is often related to the patient's occupation or hobby (e.g. teachers, singers).
* Local vocal cord disease (e.g. cysts, nodules, Reinke's oedema).
* Neoplasia – Particularly SCC of the larynx.
* Endocrine (diabetes, hypothyroidism).
* Haematological (leukaemia, lymphoma, amyloidosis).

SPECIFIC QUESTIONS

Start with an open question asking the patient to explain what changes have been noticed in his or her voice. This gives you a good opportunity to objectively assess the patient's voice.

* How long have the changes been happening for?
* Did they happen gradually or did they have a sudden onset? (Neoplasia tends to cause a gradually increasing hoarseness.)
* Is your voice getting better or worse?
* Does your voice have times when it is normal or is it always hoarse?
* Did anything bring this on? (For example, did it come on after sustained vocal use or after periods of heavy smoking?)
* Do you ever lose your voice completely?
* Have you had any recent coughs or colds? (This may be indicative of an infective laryngitis.)
* Do you clear your throat a lot?
* Do you have the feeling of catarrh or sticking phlegm?

- Do you cough a lot? Is it worse when lying down?
- Do you get symptoms of acid reflux (gastro-oesophageal reflux)? (This may overlap with LPR and predispose to pepsin-induced changes to the vocal folds.)
- Do you have a sensation of something in your throat?
- Do you have any problems swallowing? (Any problem swallowing or FOSIT should prompt further investigation, as this is a common presentation of upper aerodigestive tract tumours [*see* Section 1.15].)
- Do you have any pain in the throat or ears? (This can be primary or referred.)
- Do you have any heartburn or chest pain?
- Do you have shortness of breath or haemoptysis? (This is important, as chest disease may manifest as dysphonia due to inadequate airflow production.)
- Do you have any new lumps in the head or neck? (Lymphadenopathy can result from local disease but it can also result from lung cancer. Thyroid enlargement can also be a causative factor.)
- Screen for the patient's ideas, concerns and expectations.

PAST MEDICAL HISTORY AND GENERAL SYSTEMS REVIEW

- Are you generally a well person? (Ask specifically about weight loss, fever and malaise as signs of systemic disease.)
- Ask specifically about diabetes, thyroid disease and neurological conditions.

These can present as voice changes, although this is rarely the only symptom.

- Ask specifically about chest and heart disease, as both can cause hoarseness.
- Ask about previous thyroid or thoracic surgery, a known risk factor for recurrent laryngeal nerve damage.
- Have you had any surgery? (Any procedure under general anaesthetic may give rise to the traumatic effects of intubation.)

DRUG HISTORY

- Are you on any medications?
- Do you have any allergies to medications?

FAMILY HISTORY

- Do any conditions run in the family?

SOCIAL HISTORY

- Do you smoke or drink alcohol?
- What do you do for work? Do you have any hobbies where you shout or sing? (Ask about voice abuse, e.g. teachers, singers.)

FURTHER DISCUSSION: EXPLANATION AND PLANNING

Explain you would fully examine the head and neck and perform FNE, paying particular attention to the larynx.

You should ask the patient to read a standard paragraph or to count to 10. The voice can then be graded on the GRBAS (grade, roughness, breathiness, asthenia, strain) scale, with each characteristic given a grading between 1 and 4 (where 4 is a severe disturbance).

If the history and examination point to a functional cause, reassurance and education are important. It is advisable for the patient to avoid situations that strain the voice. A period of voice rest can be advised. General smoking and drinking advice should be given.

Most patients will get better with these lifestyle changes; however, referral to a voice therapist or specialist voice clinic is appropriate for chronic cases.

In patients describing acid reflux symptoms, LPR may account for their dysphonia. The role of LPR is poorly understood. However, in patients with reflux symptoms, a trial of PPIs and alginate solutions (which also stop pepsin and bile acid regurgitation by forming a physical barrier) is a reasonable course of action.

Surgery is appropriate for organic lesions such as polyps and for medialisation of paralysed cords. For idiopathic vocal cord palsies it is normal practice to wait at least 1 year to allow spontaneous return of normal voice.

Patients at high risk of malignancy or with lesions visible with FNE should proceed to microlaryngoscopy +/− biopsies under general anaesthetic. These patients should have an initial CXR and CT of the neck and chest.

Treatment of malignant disease will be as part of a multidisciplinary team and it will involve surgery, radiotherapy or both.

OTOLOGY

1.17   TINNITUS

A 70-year-old man comes to your outpatient clinic reporting a 10-year history of ringing in his ears, which he particularly notices when he is trying to sleep.

Tinnitus is perception of sound within the ear in the absence of any external sound. It is a very common complaint and it typically takes the form of a ringing noise. It is reported that one in three of the adult population have some tinnitus experience.

Tinnitus can be sensed in one or both ears or more non-specifically 'inside the head'. Broadly, tinnitus can be classified as objective (a sound perceived by the clinician, e.g. a bruit) or subjective (a sound only perceived by the patient). Tinnitus is subjective in the vast majority of cases.

GENERAL STRUCTURE OF THE CONSULTATION

In clinical practice, most often the only coincidental pathology is SNHL. However, it is important to differentiate these cases from cases caused by more sinister pathologies such as vestibular schwannoma or other specific otological diseases like Ménière's disease.

The pathogenesis of subjective tinnitus is far from understood. A number of models have been used to explain some of the underlying complexities. For example, one model defines an 'ignition site' caused by perturbation anywhere in the auditory system and a 'promotion site' where the initial signal is enhanced, occurring in the central auditory system. This is then overlaid with anxiety/psychosomatic effects.

Important causes of subjective tinnitus include

- Otological – Noise trauma, ear infection, otitis media, wax impaction, presbycusis/SNHL, Ménière's disease, vestibular schwannoma, other skull base tumours (e.g. glomus tympanicum)
- Medications – E.g. aspirin (not at therapeutic dose), non-steroidal anti-inflammatory drugs, ototoxic antibiotics, e.g. gentamicin, cisplatin (many other drugs list tinnitus as a side effect; however, there is scant evidence for causation for most)
- Systemic disease – Thyroid disease, vitamin B_{12} deficiency, anaemia
- Psychiatric disease – Anxiety, depression

Causes of objective tinnitus include a dehiscent jugular bulb, dural venous fistula and cartotid artery stenosis.

SPECIFIC QUESTIONS

- Ask the patient to describe the symptoms.
- How long have you experienced this?
- Is it intermittent or is it always there?
- How loud is it?
- Is it on one side or both sides? (Unilateral tinnitus requires the possibility of a retrocochlear lesion to be ruled out by intracranial imaging.)
- Is the symptom worse with noise or worse in silence?

- What is the character of the noise? (This can often be classified as pulsatile, ringing or clicking.)
- What is your hearing like? (Tinnitus is often associated with hearing loss.)
- Are you ever troubled by very loud sounds? (Hyperacusis may indicate recruitment with hearing loss.)
- Do you have any pain in the ears?
- Do you have any discharge?
- Do you have any fullness in the ear(s)?
- Do you have any vertigo or sense of imbalance? (A combination of aural fullness, hearing loss, tinnitus and vertigo may suggest the possibility of vestibular schwannoma or Ménière's disease.)
- Does it stop you sleeping? (Sleep disturbance is often reported that may exacerbate underlying anxiety and propagate the vicious cycle.)
  - Can you change the tinnitus? Modultion of tinnitus, e.g. by jaw clenching signifies somatic tinnitus.
- How is it affecting your life? Screen for signs of depression and anxiety and the patient's ideas, concerns and expectations. You should specifically explore the patient's fears of having a brain tumour. This is a common concern in the examination and in clinical practice.

PAST MEDICAL HISTORY AND GENERAL SYSTEMS REVIEW

- Do you have any other medical conditions? (Ask about general health including cardiovascular disease and diabetes.)
- Explore the patient's ideas, concerns and expectations.

DRUG HISTORY

- Are you on any medications? (A number of drugs have been associated with tinnitus including over-the-counter herbal supplements. Aspirin, antimalarials, diuretics, ototoxic antibiotics and benzodiazepines are known to be associated with SNHL and hence tinnitus.)
- Do you have any allergies to medications?

FAMILY HISTORY

- Do any conditions run in the family?

SOCIAL HISTORY

- Do you smoke or drink alcohol?
- What do you do for work?

FURTHER DISCUSSION: EXPLANATION AND PLANNING

Explain you would perform a full head and neck examination.

Otoscopy should be performed to check for obvious otological pathology and middle ear pathology including glomus tumours (pulsatile tinnitus); in this case, auscultation of the ear and neck for a bruit should be performed.

Audiometry is required to document the baseline hearing level. Plan examination of fundi for signs of raised ICP.

Formal vestibular function tests are occasionally required if there is a history of vestibular dysfunction.

Cranial nerve examination – Skull base lesions can impinge on cranial nerves as they enlarge, producing focal neurological signs.

Plan MRI of the head (with gadolinium contrast if normal renal function) if a tumour is suspected, e.g. from unilateral tinnitus, signs of raised ICP.

Without specific otological disease, surgery is not recommended (previous cochlear destruction/nerve sectioning are of limited effectiveness and offer serious risk to the patient).

Management of otological disease such as chronic suppurative otitis media (CSOM) or otosclerosis has variable outcomes on tinnitus.

If there is no organic pathology, the treatment is conservative: reassurance, counselling, CBT, tinnitus retraining therapy, white noise generators for masking, and hearing aids for SNHL. Audiology colleagues are often very helpful for managing thee patients and offering tinnitus therapy.

There is no role for medication; although a number of therapies have been tried over the years, the evidence for any particular treatment is sparse.

1.18   FACIAL WEAKNESS

A 40-year-old man is referred to your clinic with a history of a unilateral facial weakness for the last 2 days.

The facial nerve (cranial nerve VII) is derived from the second branchial arch and contains motor, sensory and parasympathetic fibres. The facial motor nucleus is in the pons.

The motor branch supplies the muscles of facial expression, buccinators, stylohyoid, stapedius, posterior belly of digastric and platysma. The sensory branch carries taste via the chorda tympani.

The parasympathetic component supplies the secretomotor function for the submandibular/sublingual salivary glands and nasal, lacrimal and palatine mucosal glands.

The nerve is classically divided into four subsections: a cerebellopontine, internal acoustic meatus, intratemporal and an extratemporal division.

Facial nerve weakness is classified on the House–Brackmann classification of facial nerve palsy (I for normal to VI for no movement).

GENERAL STRUCTURE OF THE CONSULTATION

When structuring this consultation it is important to be mindful of the anatomy of the nerve. This will help you give a logical format and ensure that possible causes are not forgotten. Facial weakness can occur with impairment at any part of the neuromuscular tract.

The most common causes of facial weakness are

- Bell's palsy (idiopathic facial nerve palsy)
- Ramsay Hunt syndrome (herpes zoster oticus)
- Neoplasia, e.g. parotid malignancy
- Trauma, e.g. birth trauma or skull base fracture
- Infection, e.g. AOM/CSOM or Lyme disease
- Congenital
- Central nervous system dysfunction, e.g. stroke

Although the differential diagnosis of a facial nerve weakness is broad, the history and examination significantly aid in diagnosis.

SPECIFIC QUESTIONS

- When did the weakness start?
- What did you first notice?
- Is it just one side or have you noticed changes to the other side?
- Did it come on suddenly or has it been coming on gradually? (The time course is not always instructive, as all causes can progress at similar rates. However, in cases that are not improving after 6 weeks, further investigation to rule out neoplasia should be undertaken.)
- Have you had any recent coughs or colds? (Post-viral facial palsy is a common cause.)
- Have you had any changes to your ears? (Ask specifically about otalgia, vesicles, hearing loss, vertigo, tinnitus and discharge. These are specific questions for associated otological disease. Possibilities that should be considered include AOM with a dehiscent facial nerve, malignant OE, cholesteatoma and skull base neoplasia.)

- Did you have any surgery to the ears?
- Have you had any trauma to your head lately? (Temporal bone fractures can compromise the nerve.)
- Have you been at depth or to high altitude recently? (Patients with a dehiscent facial nerve canal can present with facial baroparesis, which tends to be a self-resolving neuropraxia.)
- Have you noticed any other weaknesses or sensory disturbances in the rest of the body? (Other central nervous system [CNS] pathology, e.g. multiple sclerosis or stroke, should always be considered.)

PAST MEDICAL HISTORY AND GENERAL SYSTEMS REVIEW

- Do you have any other conditions? (Ask specifically about hypertension and diabetes.)
- Have you ever had a cancer or tumour diagnosed? (Metastatic disease from other head and neck primary sites is possible.)
- Any family history of similar occurrences?

DRUG HISTORY

- Are you on any medications?
- Do you have any allergies to medications?

FAMILY HISTORY

- Do any conditions run in the family?

SOCIAL HISTORY

- Do you smoke or drink alcohol?
- What do you do for work?
- Have you been travelling recently? (For example, have you travelled to areas where Lyme disease is endemic?)

FURTHER DISCUSSION: EXPLANATION AND PLANNING

Explain you would perform a full examination of the facial nerve and grade the weakness (e.g. using the House–Brackmann scale).

The weakness should be classified into upper motor neuron (UMN) or lower motor neuron (LMN) lesion. Bicortical representation means there is forehead sparing in a UMN lesion, e.g. with a stroke. With an LMN palsy, e.g. Bell's palsy, there will be weakness in all divisions of the face.

Plan a full examination of the ipsilateral ear and mastoid.

Plan a full cranial nerve examination; check the cranial nerve V in particular, as paraesthesia or pain in this distribution can be a rare sign of vestibular schwannoma. Examine the cerebellum including gait, Romberg and Unterberger tests and look for dysdiadochokinesia and past pointing.

Plan a flexible nasendoscopy to rule out a nasopharyngeal cancer. These can involve any of the cranial nerves. By this stage in progression it is very likely that other, lower cranial nerves will also be compromised.

Plan a full examination of the parotid gland to rule out a parotid tumour. A parotid mass with facial nerve palsy is suggestive of malignancy, e.g. mucoepidermoid, adenoid cystic subtypes.

PTA should be performed to document the baseline hearing level.

Treatment: first, educate about eye protection. This is particularly important at night, as corneal drying can result in corneal ulceration and, ultimately, blindness.

If an obvious cause is found, such as parotid mass, then manage this appropriately, e.g. perform fine needle aspiration (FNA) for histology.

Blood tests, e.g. Lyme disease serology, should only be performed if indicated from the history.

In the absence of an obvious diagnosis it is appropriate to make an initial diagnosis of Bell's palsy. A 7- to 10-day reducing dose of corticosteroid improves prognosis. Antivirals have not been shown to improve recovery but are still used by many clinicians. With treatment 94% of those affected show complete resolution of symptoms at 9 months.

Ramsay Hunt syndrome (varicella zoster infection manifesting as facial weakness and otic vesicles) is routinely treated with a course of aciclovir and reducing corticosteroids.

The patient should be followed up in 3–4 weeks. Lack of recovery may indicate the need for further investigation to rule out neoplasia (most often MRI of the course of the facial nerve).

1.19   ADULT WITH ITCHY, PAINFUL EAR

A 50-year-old man has been referred to the ENT casualty clinic with a 2-week history of a painful and itchy left ear. He has tried a number of ear drops from his general practitioner (GP).

The painful, itchy ear is a very common presentation in ENT outpatient clinics most commonly caused by OE. Routinely, microsuction, symptom control and topical antibiotic therapy are all that is required. However, it is important to remember more sinister causes such as necrotising otitis externa (NOE, a life-threatening spreading osteomyelitis of the skull base).

GENERAL STRUCTURE OF THE CONSULTATION

The most common cause for this presentation in the casualty clinic is OE.

This is defined as an inflammation of the auricle and/or external auditory canal (EAC) up to the medial surface of the TM. It is typically caused by infection, allergy or trauma.

OE can be both acute (under 3 weeks) and chronic (over 3 weeks). The ear canal is often full of debris and is inflamed and narrowed. The presence of inflammatory exudates in the canal can lead to a vicious cycle of exudate, inflammation and pain that is difficult to break. Initially only limited examination may be possible.

SPECIFIC QUESTIONS

- What symptoms are you getting? (Ask specifically about otalgia, discharge, aural fullness and vertigo. If they are getting discharge, ask about the colour, consistency, smell and amount.)
- How long have you had the symptoms?
- What treatment have you received?
- Do you have trouble with the ears frequently and, if so, for how long?
- Do you often get the ears wet? Are you involved in swimming or surfing? (These are typical risk factors for OE.)
- Do you use ear buds to clean your ears or routinely use in-the-ear devices (such as hearing aids or earphones)?
- Have you had any trauma to the ears recently?
- Do you have any allergies? (Patients can develop a type IV hypersensitivity reaction to metals found in earrings such as nickel. Unfortunately, patients can also develop allergies to antibiotics, e.g. topical neomycin.)
- Do you have any other weaknesses or changes in sensation in your body? (It is important to rule out focal neurology, e.g. cranial nerve VII palsy, and severe pain may be indicative of NOE.)
- Do you have any pain in the teeth, tonsils, jaw, throat, face or neck? (Pathology outside the ear can be both a cause and a consequence of otalgia due to referred pain.)

PAST MEDICAL HISTORY AND GENERAL SYSTEMS REVIEW

- Do you have any other medical conditions? (Ask specifically about diabetes, which is a risk factor for both benign and NOE, and skin conditions such as dermatitis and eczema.)

DRUG HISTORY

- Are you on any medications? (Most patients will have been started on topical antibiotics by the time they are seen in clinic. It is important to find out the type and course length in order to guide appropriate therapy.)
- Do you have any allergies to medications?

FAMILY HISTORY

- Do any conditions run in the family?

SOCIAL HISTORY

- Do you smoke or drink alcohol?
- What do you do for work?

FURTHER DISCUSSION: EXPLANATION AND PLANNING

Explain you would perform a full examination of both ears.

Examine for surrounding cellulitis and lymphadenopathy.

Examine mastoids and note any erythema or pinna protrusion. This may signify mastoiditis, although this is extremely rare in adults.

Perform otoscopy – Often the canal is filled with debris, which will need to be cleared under microscopic guidance. Middle ear discharge (with underlying perforation) is normally mucoid and can be pulsatile due to middle ear vasculature. It is important to try to completely clear the EAC and to visualise the status of the TM. The quality and consistency of the discharge may signify the infective organism, e.g. offensive, green discharge is typical with *Pseudomonas* infection. Similarly, it may be possible to visualise fungal hyphae.

Often the EAC is inflamed and narrowed and only minimal suction clearance can be performed. This necessitates the placement of an aural wick for instilment of topical antibiotics. The patient should then be seen in 3–4 days' time for removal of the wick and further attempts at suction clearance.

If otoscopy is normal then it is worth considering the possibility of referred pain (*see* Section 1.22).

If granulation tissue is seen in the canal, it is prudent to obtain CT imaging, particularly in elderly, immunocompromised patients. NOE may present with severe otalgia and/or cranial nerve palsies, depending on the extent of the disease. These patients need long-term intravenous antibiotics and, rarely, surgical debridement.

The cornerstones of OE treatment are aural toilet, analgesia and topical antibiotics.

Advise the patient on aural hygiene – Particularly regarding keeping the ears dry when showering. (Vaseline-soaked cotton wool can be useful for this.)

Consider topical antibiotics including Sofradex, Otosporin, Otomize or antifungals, e.g. clotrimazole solution.

In ongoing infections, a swab should be taken for culture and sensitivity, and antibiotics should be chosen on the basis of these.

Acetic acid (Ear Calm) can be useful in controlling symptoms.

There is rarely a need to use systemic antibiotics unless the patient presents with cellulitis or NOE or is immunocompromised.

1.20   ADULT WITH NON-ACUTE HEARING LOSS

A 54-year-old man is brought to the ENT clinic by his wife who is fed up having to shout to be heard at home.

Hearing loss is extremely common in the general adult population. It can range from extremely mild to profound loss with subsequent impact on social functioning and quality of life. Approximately 10% of the adult population has some degree of hearing loss; however, this rises to 35% in the age group over 65 years. Hearing loss can result from impairment to any part of the auditory pathway, from the auricle to the CNS. Gradual hearing loss in the adult tends to be sensorineural in origin resulting from lesions of the inner ear or vestibulocochlear nerve (cranial nerve VIII).

GENERAL STRUCTURE OF THE CONSULTATION

This is a common presentation in ENT clinic. The key to making a diagnosis is in the history. The majority of these patients will have idiopathic SNHL. However, it is worth remembering other identifiable causes, e.g. infections, neoplasia, trauma, neurological reasons, metabolic reasons, toxicity and autoimmune reasons.

SPECIFIC QUESTIONS

* What have you noticed about your hearing?
* How severe is the loss and how is it affecting your day-to-day activities?
* Did it come on gradually or suddenly? (Try to ascertain the exact circumstances when the hearing loss was noticed.) Sudden sensorineural hearing loss is a medical emergency (see Section 1.21).
* How was your hearing before?
* Is it one ear or both ears?
* Have you had problems with your ears in the past? (Ask specifically about tinnitus, fullness, dizziness, pain, discharge and wax problems.)
* Have you had any recent coughs or colds? (These may predispose to OME.)
* Have you had any recent chest infections, sinusitis or kidney problems? (This screens for autoimmune conditions and granulomatous disease that can present with hearing loss and systemic symptoms.)
* Do you have any problems with your nose? (Ask about discharge, epistaxis and obstruction. This screens for PNS lesions that are associated with OME.)
* Do you have any weaknesses or changes in sensation? (Cranial nerve lesions are a feature of advanced neoplasia.)
* Did you have any recent trauma to your head? (Temporal bone fractures can disrupt the auditory pathways.)

PAST MEDICAL HISTORY AND GENERAL SYSTEMS REVIEW

* Do you have any other medical conditions? (Ask specifically about autoimmune conditions and weight loss, fevers, lethargy, malaise (with neoplasia and granulomatous disease), hypertension, hyperlipidaemia and exposure to infectious agents, e.g. syphilis or HIV.

DRUG HISTORY

- Are you on any medications? (A number of drugs are associated with hearing loss, particularly aminoglycoside antibiotics, platinum chemotherapeutic agents and loop diuretics.)
- Do you have any allergies to medications?

FAMILY HISTORY

- Do any conditions run in the family? (Hearing loss may have a genetic basis.)

SOCIAL HISTORY

- Do you smoke or drink alcohol?
- What do you do for work? (Ask about noise exposure).

FURTHER DISCUSSION: EXPLANATION AND PLANNING

Explain you would perform a full examination of both ears including otoscopy, PTA and tympanogram.

If findings are suggestive of OME, examine the PNS to rule out any neoplasia, e.g. nasopharyngeal carcinoma.

If there are other 'red flag' symptoms such as unilateral hearing loss or tinnitus, vertigo or vestibular symptoms, then intracranial imaging may be appropriate.

Consider investigation for autoimmune/granulomatous disease, depending on history.

Most hearing loss in adults will be SNHL with underlying genetic aetiology. Noise-induced hearing loss and presbycusis are also often implicated – consider referral to audiology care for hearing device assessment. Otosclerosis is the commonest cause of progressive hearing loss in young adults and this can be managed with either hearing aids or stapes surgery.

1.21   ADULT WITH SUDDEN HEARING LOSS

A 29-year-old man is referred by his GP with a history of unilateral hearing loss for 72 hours.

GENERAL STRUCTURE OF THE CONSULTATION

A sudden SNHL is defined as a sensorineural loss of 30 dB or more, over at least three contiguous audiometric frequencies that develops over 3 days or less in an ear with previously normal hearing or a decrease in hearing in an ear with a pre-existing loss. It is worth noting conductive losses can present similarly. The majority of cases are idiopathic; however, there are some important treatable causes that must be ruled out.

SPECIFIC QUESTIONS

- How did you notice the hearing loss?
- How severe is it?
- Did the hearing loss come on gradually or suddenly? (Many patients notice hearing loss when they wake up in the morning or when trying to use the telephone with that ear.)
- How was your hearing before? (Hearing loss can occur in previously normal ears, ears with a pre-existing hearing impairment or as part of a disorder with fluctuating hearing levels, such as Ménière's disease.)
- Is the hearing loss in one ear or in both ears? (3% of vestibular schwannomas present with sudden hearing loss.)
- Do you have any other symptoms? (Ask specifically about vertigo, tinnitus, wax problems and discharge.)
- Screen for the patient's ideas, concerns and expectations.

PAST MEDICAL HISTORY AND GENERAL SYSTEMS REVIEW

- Do you have any other medical conditions? (Systemic diseases including multiple sclerosis, antiphospholipid syndrome and autoimmune diseases could theoretically present initially with sudden hearing loss. Ask about neurological conditions – such as drop attacks, transient loss of consciousness, neck pain, weaknesses, paraesthesias, vertigo and double vision – as these can be the presentation of vertebrobasilar insufficiency.)
- Have you been diagnosed with a cancer or tumour in the past? (Sudden hearing loss can be caused post irradiation and as an effect of chemotherapy agents such as cisplatin.)
- Have you been exposed to any loud sounds or any recent head trauma? (A perilymph fistula should be considered if there is a history of pressure changes and sudden hearing loss associated with a positive fistula test [nystagmus when applying manual pressure to the ipsilateral tragus].)

DRUG HISTORY

- Are you on any medications? (It is important to take a full drug history, as there are some commonly used ototoxic medications – particularly, platinum-based chemotherapy, aminoglycoside antibiotics, salicylates and loop diuretics.)
- Do you have any allergies to medications?

FAMILY HISTORY

- Do any conditions run in the family?

SOCIAL HISTORY

- Have you been travelling recently? (Ask about foreign travel and travel to areas with endemic Lyme disease.)
- Ascertain a sexual history. HIV and syphilis are associated with sudden hearing loss.

FURTHER DISCUSSION: EXPLANATION AND PLANNING

Explain you would perform a full ear examination including otoscopy to exclude any conductive losses such as OME or wax.

Plan a full examination of cranial nerves – hearing loss with other focal neurology may suggest a vascular/neoplastic origin, e.g. paraesthesia in distribution of cranial nerve V with vestibular schwannomas or diplopia with cranial nerve VI involvement.

Perform a fistula test if the history is suggestive of a perilymphatic fistula. Perform PTA/tympanometry to get an objective measure of the hearing loss.

Blood tests should be ordered in correspondence with the clinical history and examination findings. For example, HbA1c in suspected diabetes or FBC, ESR or autoimmune antibody screen if autoimmune pathology is suspected.

In unilateral hearing loss, gadolinium contrast MRI is the most useful examination of the internal acoustic meatus for retrocochlear causes.

Treatment is decided on the basis of clinical findings. There is no obvious cause in the majority of cases. This should be explained to the patient.

Numerous treatment regimens including steroids, plasma expanders, aciclovir and carbogen have been tried; however, the evidence remains inconclusive.

A number of studies have pointed to the benefit of a short, high-dose regimen of oral corticosteroids for sudden unilateral hearing loss (a commonly used protocol is 1 mg/kg up to 60mg prednisolone for 7 days). Patients should be informed of the risk involved with taking steroids, such as disturbed sleep and gastric ulceration. Intratympanic steroids may be considered in those where systemic therapy is contraindicated or if there has been no improvement with systemic therapy.

Arrange to follow up with the patient in 4–6 weeks to repeat hearing tests and to monitor progress.

In cases where there is no improvement, hearing aids may be considered, particularly in bilateral cases (often no treatment is required in unilateral cases).

Patients must be informed that they need to seek urgent medical attention if they experience hearing loss in the contralateral ear, as immediate treatment is very likely to be warranted.

1.22 OTALGIA

A 30-year-old man is referred to the ENT clinic with a 3-month history of left-sided ear pain.

GENERAL STRUCTURE OF THE CONSULTATION

Otalgia is a complicated presenting complaint as there are a numerous possible causes. Pain can be of otological (outer, middle or inner ear) or non-otological origin. Careful history taking and examination is required.

SPECIFIC QUESTIONS

- When did the pain start?
- Is it getting better or worse?
- What makes it better or worse?
- Do you notice any other symptoms with the pain?
- Do you have any problems with your teeth? TMJ dysfunction and dental pathology can present with otalgia.
- Do you have any problems with your nose? (Ask specifically about rhinorrhea, obstruction, catarrh and post-nasal drip, as rhinosinusitis associated with eustachian tube dysfunction can present as otalgia.)
- Have you had any recent coughs and colds? (Odynophagia with referred otalgia is commonly associated with infections of the upper aerodigestive tract such as tonsillitis and pharyngitis, but also with neoplastic disease.)
- Do you get heartburn or reflux? (Reflux can be associated with otalgia.)
- Do you have any pain or limitation in movement of the neck? (This can imply referred otalgia is due to the irritation of the upper cervical nerve roots.)

PAST MEDICAL HISTORY AND GENERAL SYSTEMS REVIEW

- Do you have any other conditions? (Ask specifically about hypertension, diabetes.)
- Have you been diagnosed with a cancer or tumour in the past? (Metastatic disease from other head and neck primary sites is possible.)

DRUG HISTORY

- Are you on any medications?
- Do you have any allergies to medications?

FAMILY HISTORY

- Do any conditions run in the family?

SOCIAL HISTORY

- Do you smoke or drink alcohol?
- What do you do for work?

FURTHER DISCUSSION: EXPLANATION AND PLANNING

Explain you would perform a full examination of the ear.

Full examination of the cranial nerves is very important, as other neurological signs may be indicative of a space-occupying lesion, for example, lesions of the petrous apex V/VI deficit, lower cranial nerve lesions in metastatic tumours of the pharynx/larynx and VII nerve palsy in parotid gland malignancy.

Examine the dentition and temporomandibular joints.

Examine the cervical spine for joint tenderness, neck movements and muscle spasms.

Other investigations include orthopantogram (dental X-ray), barium swallow, panendoscopy and biopsy.

In patients with risk factors or when clinically suspected, MRI of the head and neck may be indicated to rule out malignancy, particularly in areas difficult to detect clinically such as the tongue base and tonsil.

1.23 DIZZINESS

A 28-year-old woman attends the ENT clinic complaining of feeling dizzy.

GENERAL STRUCTURE OF THE CONSULTATION

The complexity of the vestibular system coupled with the often non-specific symptoms of the patients make evaluating the dizzy patient a difficult consultation. However, with a careful history it is possible to differentiate the important causes and often to provide appropriate therapy. Ultimately, you must distinguish between true vertigo and imbalance, and peripheral from central causes of vertigo.

SPECIFIC QUESTIONS

- Please explain to me what is happening when you are dizzy. (Differentiate between true vertigo ['the room spins'], disequilibrium sense of imbalance presyncope [the feeling of faintness] and general non-specific 'light-headedness'. In dizzy patients without true vertigo, an underlying medical cause such as cardiac arrhythmia needs to be ruled out. For the purposes of the ENT clinic, we focus on the patients with true vertigo.)
- Tell me about the first time you became dizzy. (Allow the patient to speak without interrupting her. This will elucidate the time course of the onset of the dizziness and will suggest a cause of acute vestibular failure that may not be clear from the rest of the history.)
- Are you always dizzy or does it come in episodes?
- Tell me more about an episode.
- How often do the episodes come and how long do they last? (Short, self-terminating episodes that are positionally determined [e.g. turning over in bed] suggest benign paroxysmal positional vertigo [BPPV]. Longer episodes are suggestive of vestibular failure [e.g. vestibular neuronitis]. Continued vertigo is suggestive of central causes, e.g. multiple sclerosis.)
- Is there anything you can do to make it better? (Ask if visual fixation improves the vertigo. A peripheral cause for vertigo is improved, while a central vertigo is unaffected.)
- Is there anything you have noticed that brings on the vertigo? (Ask about characteristic head positions for BPPV or the occurrence of vertigo with loud sounds [Tullio's phenomenon] that may indicate an underlying superior canal dehiscence.)
- Have you noticed associated symptoms? (Particularly, enquire about hearing loss, tinnitus, aural discharge. A presentation of episodic low-tone hearing loss, aural fullness, tinnitus and vertigo is pathognomic of Ménière's disease. Vertigo with 'aura' such as visual or olfactory disturbance, or sensitivity to lights/sounds with a history of migraine is suggestive of vestibular migraine. Vertigo with asymmetric hearing loss and/or tinnitus could be a result of a vestibular schwannoma (a rare presenting symptom).)
- Were you unwell before the first episode of dizziness? (Viral infections predispose to vestibular neuronitis/labyrinthitis.)

PAST MEDICAL HISTORY AND GENERAL SYSTEMS REVIEW

- Do you have any other medical conditions? (Ask about general health including cardiovascular disease, diabetes, eye problems and mobility or joint problems – these conditions often manifest as imbalance.)
- Have you had any recent trauma to the head? (Temporal bone fractures can involve the vestibular system.)
- Have you had any previous surgery to the ears?
- Explore the patient's ideas, concerns and expectations. Specifically, explore the patient's fear around the possibility of brain tumours. This is very likely to be what the patient is worried about.

DRUG HISTORY

- Are you on any medications? (Ask about use of antibiotics. For example, gentamicin is known to be toxic to both the vestibular and the cochlear systems. Antihypertensives cause positional hypotension, an important cause of disequilibrium particularly in the elderly. It is important that multiple medications and multiple co-morbidities in the elderly lead to multifactorial dizziness.)
- Do you have any allergies to medications?

FAMILY HISTORY

- Do any conditions run in the family? (Ask about Meniere's disease.)

SOCIAL HISTORY

- Do you smoke or drink alcohol? (Ask about relation of these activities to the symptoms.)
- What do you do for work? (Ask about the effect of the symptoms on the patient's ability to do his or her job safely. This is important if the patient drives for a living.)
- Ask about stress. (Vertigo can be a psychogenic condition that improves with stress management techniques.)
- Are you currently driving? (The patient may need to contact the Driver and Vehicle Licensing Agency for advice as to whether it is appropriate to continue to drive.)

FURTHER DISCUSSION: EXPLANATION AND PLANNING

Explain that you will need to examine the patient's ears, eyes and sense of balance with some simple tests.

Lying and standing blood pressures should be taken. A significant postural drop may indicate the true cause of the patient's symptoms.

Perform a standard examination of the ear. This is to rule out any middle ear disease, e.g. OME or cholesteatoma. Perform a fistula test.

Assess for the presence of nystagmus. A horizontal nystagmus is typical of a peripheral vertigo. Vertical nystagmus indicates a central cause. The direction of the nystagmus is classically described in terms of the direction of the fast phase.

Perform a head thrust test. In acute vestibular failure, the vestibulo-ocular response fails and fixation is lost requiring a corrective saccade.

Perform a full examination of all other cranial nerves. Gross signs are often obvious but subtler signs, such as a V nerve palsy manifesting as a loss of corneal reflex with a vestibular schwannoma, are easier to miss.

Perform balance tests – Unterberger and Romberg tests can reveal gross derangements in equilibrium, but they are not specific in differentiating central from peripheral lesions.

Perform a Dix–Hallpike procedure for BPPV (there are numerous videos available online for more information on this procedure).

Inform the patient that you will formally assess his or her hearing with a pure-tone audiogram.

Imaging is indicated in patients with unilateral symptoms, e.g. vertigo with unilateral tinnitus or SNHL. In most units the imaging of choice is MRI, primarily to exclude vestibular schwannomas but also to examine the CNS for other conditions, such as brainstem plaques in multiple sclerosis.

Other tests such as the caloric test are not often performed in routine clinical practice.

Treatment will depend on the underlying condition. Patients with acute vestibular failure should be reassured and informed that their condition will improve naturally. They should be directed to a trustworthy balance information source for vestibular rehabilitation exercises if the balance disorder continues. Vestibular sedatives may be of use in the acute phase.

In patients with a positive Dix–Hallpike result, an Epley procedure can be performed in clinic. This procedure has a high success rate in BPPV and it can be repeated. Patients can also be taught how to perform the procedure at home. (There are a number of training aids available, e.g. DizzyFIX.)

The management of Ménière's disease follows a step-wise approach. Low risk interventions include the adoption of a low-sodium diet. Caffeine and tobacco have also been suggested as exacerbating factors. There is equivocal evidence for treatment with diuretics. Crises can be treated with vestibular sedatives and antiemetics. There is good evidence that intratympanic steroids reduce the number of episodes. In severe cases, the patient may opt for ablative therapy (intratympanic gentamicin, endolymphatic sac surgery, labyrinthectomy, vestibular nerve section).

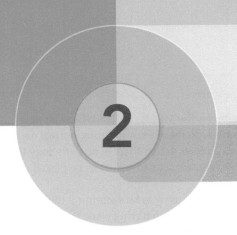

Examination Stations

2

The MRCS (ENT) OSCE examination demands a fluent and confident approach to the basic ear, nose and throat (ENT), head and neck examination. It is important to have a logical system for examining the ear, nose and neck, as these are most commonly tested in the examination.

Marks in the examination are primarily given for the form and comprehensiveness of the examination rather than for the signs elicited. You might find it helpful to talk through what you are doing and what you have found as you go. Some examiners will require you to do this, although most stay relatively passive and allow you to continue with the examination at your own pace.

The general examination schema learnt in medical school – inspection, palpation and auscultation – holds true here. This needs to be modified for the head and neck examination, as palpation and auscultation, whilst important, play smaller roles than in other body systems.

General rules for examinations include the following:

- Always introduce yourself and gain consent and cooperation of the patient.

A good opening may be: 'Hello, I am Dr Jones. Would it be OK if I examined your ears and hearing?'

- Always enquire whether the patient is currently in any pain. It is not good practice to cause patients pain in examinations or in clinical practice.

Tips for success in the examination stations:

- Design a scheme for examining the ear, nose and neck. Make sure that it has a logical order, covers all the important areas and that you can remember it.
- Practise your schemes at every opportunity. You do not always need patients with clinical signs for this.
- Recognise that in the examination you will be feeling nervous and stressed.

The more practice you do, the less nervy you will be when it comes to the examination. If you do forget something it is very rarely 'fatal', as you will have picked up plenty of marks elsewhere.

- Before and after you touch any patient, use the alcohol gel provided. There are lots of easy marks going for this.
- Make sure you are bare below the elbows.
- Stay calm – Things are just easier that way.

DOI: 10.1201/b23029-2

2.1 EXAMINATION OF THE EAR

This is an important examination scheme to master for the MRCS (ENT) OSCE. Get practising – repetition is most definitely the key to success. Remember, examining normal ears
is beneficial, as it makes detecting pathology much easier. Often there is no pathology to
see in the examination; however, the actors often fabricate a hearing loss to be picked up
using the objective tests described in this section.

Introduce yourself to the patient. Explain that you are going to be examining their ears
and hearing: 'Hello, I am Dr Jones. I understand you have been having some trouble with
your ears. Would it be OK if I could examine your ears and hearing?'

Clean your hands with the alcohol gel.

Tell the patient that you will be explaining to him or her what you are doing as you go
along, but let the patient know they can ask if he or she has any questions. You may or
may not be asked by the examiner to present your findings, but the focus is primarily on
procedure and completeness rather than on the findings themselves.

Ask which is the patient's 'better' ear.

Ask if the patient is currently in any pain. This is extremely important. If the patient
indicates he or she has pain from one ear then it should be examined with care.

Test your otoscope to check that it is working and then commence inspection of the
better ear (using the light from the otoscope) (Figures 2.1–2.3).

Areas to look at are as follows:

- Pinna (scars, quality of cartilage, active infections, compare symmetry with the
  other side)
- Mastoid (move the pinna forwards, asking again about pain)
- Preauricular area (look for pits, sinuses, fistulae)
- Conchal bowl

Now change the otoscope tip and proceed with examining the other ear and make a comparison between them.

Now proceed to examine the external auditory canal (EAC) and tympanic membrane
(TM) with the otoscope (held in the same hand as the ear you are examining, between
the thumb and forefinger). For this you will need to pull the pinna posterosuperiorly to

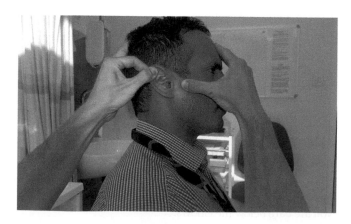

Figure 2.1 Examining the ear, pulling the pinna posterosuperiorly.

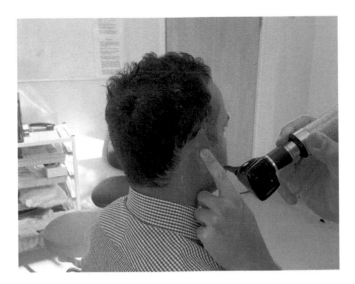

Figure 2.2 Examining the mastoid.

straighten the canal with the other hand. Choose the largest speculum that fits into the canal to give the best view of the TM (**Figures** 2.4 and 2.5).

You should use the little finger of the hand holding the otoscope to brace against the cheek of the patient; this should stop any damage to the ear if the patient makes any sudden movement.

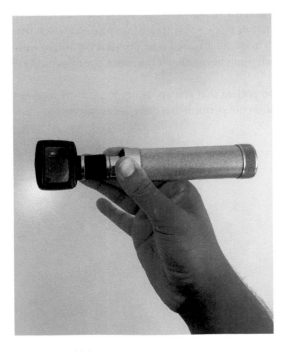

Figure 2.3 The correct way to hold the otoscope.

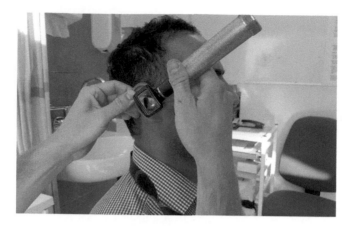

Figure 2.4 Examining the ear using the otoscope.

Be gentle with the otoscope. Make sure when you are moving it around in the EAC that your movements are slow and considered, otherwise you will cause the patient pain. In the examination the 'patient' will have had his or her ears examined a number of times before, hence their tolerance to any sudden movements is quite low.

Areas to comment on (**Figure 2.6**):

- EAC (look for discharge, bony swellings)
- Pars tensa (any perforations, retraction pockets, ossicles – particularly the lateral process and handle of malleus and long process of incus, presence of grommets)
- Pars flaccida (attic retraction pockets, cholesteatoma)

At this point, indicate to the examiner that you would usually perform pneumatic otoscopy to assess the mobility of the TM.

Next, perform the fistula test – Apply tragal pressure and watch the eyes for nystagmus with a fast phase away from the diseased side. This test is positive with a lateral semicircular canal fistula. This step can be omitted if the rubric specifies not to examine the balance system.

Next, explain to the patient that you are going to perform some tests of their hearing. (NB: These tests are often not performed if there is easy access to an audiology department

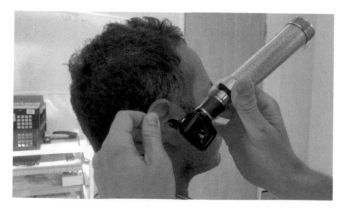

Figure 2.5 Using the otoscope, pulling the ear posterosuperiorly.

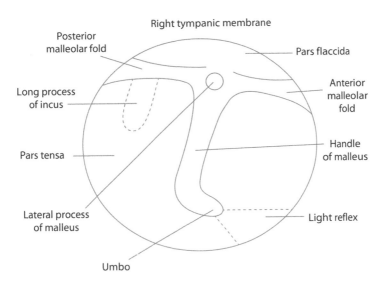

Right tympanic membrane

Posterior malleolar fold

Pars flaccida

Long process of incus

Anterior malleolar fold

Pars tensa

Handle of malleus

Lateral process of malleus

Light reflex

Umbo

Figure 2.6 A stylised version of the otoscopic view of the TM.

that can perform an audiogram; however, these tests remain useful when audiology is not available.)

First, perform a free field test of the patient's hearing (Figures 2.7 and 2.8).

The non-test ear is masked with tragal pressure and the patient's eyes are shielded to prevent any visual stimulus. Do not place your arm across the face of the patient when masking the contralateral ear. It is far nicer for the patient to occlude the ear from behind his or her head.

You will then whisper three two-syllable words or bi-digit numbers from 60 cm from the test ear. If the patient gets two out of these three correct then the hearing level is 12 dB or better.

If there is no accurate response, use a conversational voice (48 dB or worse) or a loud voice (76 dB or worse).

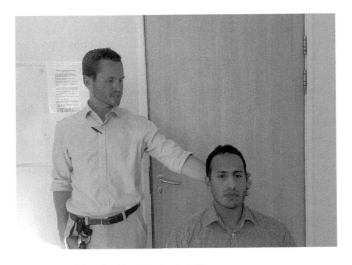

Figure 2.7 Performance of free field hearing test at 60 cm.

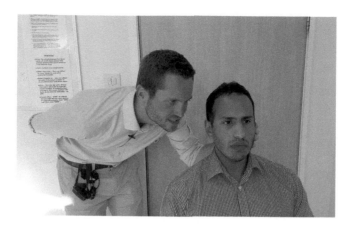

Figure 2.8 Performance of free field hearing test at 15 cm.

You can then move closer and repeat the test at 15 cm. Here the thresholds are 34 dB for a whisper and 56 dB for a conversational voice.

Next, perform Rinne and Weber tests. There will be a number of tuning forks laid out on the examination table. Always choose the 512 Hz fork (and make sure the examiner has seen you do this!). This gives the best balance between time of decay and tactile vibration (ideally, you want a fork that has a long period of decay and cannot be detected by vibration sensation).

Explain to the patient that you are going to be testing his or her hearing using the tuning forks.

Perform Weber test first, by placing a 512 Hz tuning fork in the midline forehead or the vertex. The tuning fork should be set in motion by striking it on your knee (not on the patient's knee or a table). Ask the patient whether he or she hears it loudest in the right, the left or the middle and note the result.

Next, perform Rinne test. Place a vibrating 512 Hz tuning fork firmly on the test ear mastoid process (apply pressure to the opposite side of the head to make sure the contact is firm, ideally from behind so you are not shielding the patient's eyes with your hands, as many patients find this claustrophobic). It is very important that the fork goes on to the mastoid process. It is surprising the number of people who do not perform this correctly. If you are unsure, it is wise to get one of your consultants to show you how best to do this. The examiners will certainly check the fork is correctly placed.

This tests the bone conduction. Next, place the tuning fork in front of the test ear with the tuning fork's tines perpendicular to the head, hence testing air conduction. Ask the patient which one he or she heard loudest and take note of the result.

A positive Rinne test result is NORMAL, where the air conduction is heard better than the bone conduction. This is unusual for a medical sign, where the positive sign is usually pathological. This can lead to some confusion. Normal hearing will have a positive Rinne test result in both ears and Weber test will be central (Figures 2.9–2.11).

You should present the findings to the examiner as you detected them and then interpret the findings to give a diagnosis if there is any hearing loss (Table 2.1).

This completes the examination of the ear for the purpose of the MRCS (ENT) OSCE.

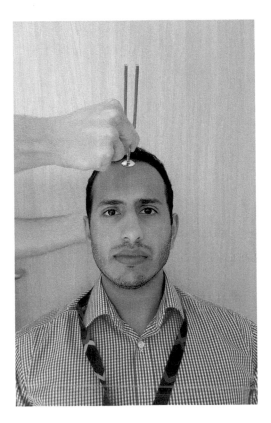

Figure 2.9 Weber test.

To complete your examination, tell the examiner you would like to examine all the cranial nerves, paying particular attention to the facial nerve. Any facial nerve weakness should be graded on the House–Brackmann scale (I–VI). You would also like to examine the post-nasal space (PNS) with a rigid endoscope, paying particular attention to the openings of the eustachian tubes, where nasopharyngeal carcinomas can arise.

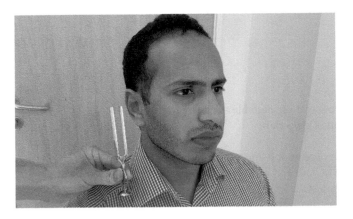

Figure 2.10 Rinne test.

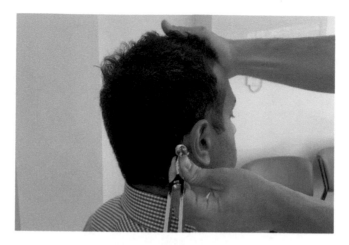

Figure 2.11 Rinne test with tuning fork on mastoid process.

Table 2.1 Findings from Rinne and Weber Tests

	Weber lateralises left	Weber lateralises right
Rinne positive both ears AC > BC	Sensorineural loss in right	Sensorineural loss in left
Rinne negative left BC > AC	Conductive loss in left	Sensorineural loss in left
Rinne negative right BC > AC	Sensorineural loss in right	Conductive loss in right

Note: AC, air conduction; BC, bone conduction.

You would also send the patient for formal audiological examination including pure-tone audiometry and tympanometry.

Thank the patient for his or her cooperation and use the alcohol gel as you leave.

EXAMINATION PEARL

Remember the four Fs, which are easy to forget in the ear exam:

Fields, Forks, Fistula, Facial nerve

EXAMPLE EAR EXAMINATION MARK SCHEME (EACH POINT SCORED TO A MAXIMUM OF FOUR POINTS)

- Introduction
- Consent, cooperation, suitable exposure
- Explanation of procedure
- Reassurance
- Correct use of otoscope (including checking it works)
- Inspection of both ears including EACs/TMs
- Tuning fork tests
- Free field hearing tests
- Fistula test
- Suggestion of extra test (cranial nerves, audio, balance system)

2.2   EXAMINATION OF THE NOSE

Introduce yourself and explain to the patient that you are going to be examining his or her nose: 'Hello, I am Dr Jones. Would it be OK if I could examine your nose and sinuses?'

Ask if the patient currently has any pain in the nose or face. Proceed with care if the patient indicates that he or she currently has tender areas.

Sit facing the patient with your knees together and to one side of the patient's knees. It is not pleasant for the patient to be 'straddled'.

Start by applying gel in your hands and then inspect the nose from the front while seated. Then you can stand and examine the nose from above, below and each side.

Areas to comment on are as follows:

- Nasal dorsum (saddling, erythema, scars, dorsal hump)
- Tip (any depression, ptosis, over-projection)
- Columella (gently elevate the tip to check for columella dislocation)

Inspect the face, commenting particularly on the presence of any rash (infection, autoimmune disease) (Figures 2.12 and 2.13).

Next, take the Thudicum speculum and carefully examine each side of the nose in turn (Figure 2.14). Make sure you are familiar with how to hold the speculum. The correct method is slightly counter-intuitive but allows the best visualisation of the nasal mucosa. Insert your index finger into the bend of the speculum and support it above with the thumb. The middle and ring fingers are used to manipulate the tines of the speculum. You are effectively looking through the gap between these two fingers.

Areas to comment on include

- Septum (perforations, deviations, mucosal damage, areas of cautery)
- Lateral wall (size of turbinates, polyps)

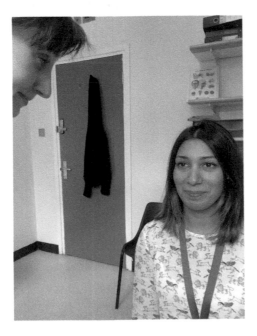

Figure 2.12 Examining the nose, inspection.

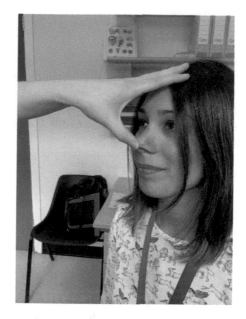

Figure 2.13 Examining the nasal vestibules with columella retraction.

Next, perform an examination of the nasal airflow by asking the patient to exhale while holding a Lack's metallic tongue depressor under the nose. Assess the pattern of fogging on the depressor.

Ask the patient to sniff in and watch for evidence of vestibular collapse.

If there is any nasal obstruction, perform Cottle's test by applying lateral pressure to the cheek at the side of the nose to see whether this improves the nasal airway (a positive Cottle's test indicates nasal valve stenosis) (Figure 2.15).

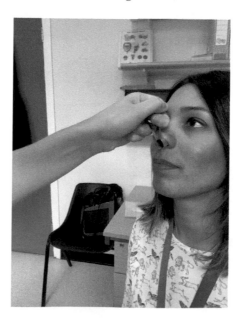

Figure 2.14 Use of the Thudicum speculum.

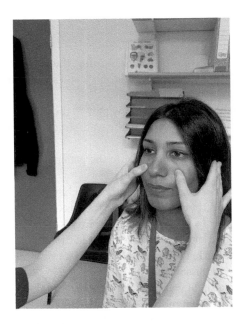

Figure 2.15 Performance of Cottle's test.

Examine the oropharynx, soft palate and upper teeth.

Suggest to the examiner that you would like to examine the nose and PNS using the rigid endoscope. Check the posterior end of the septum, the turbinates, the eustachian tube orifices and the fossae of Rosenmüller (this is where nasopharyngeal carcinomas can hide). There may be an endoscope and a manikin for you to demonstrate this on (*see* Section 2.5).

Tell the examiner you would like to assess the patient's sense of smell using the University of Pennsylvania Smell Identification Test (UPSIT). Explain that you would perform an examination of the neck for the presence of lymphadenopathy, particularly of the submandibular and jugulodigastric nodes (*see* Section 2.3). You will not be expected to perform a neck examination in a nose examination station.

Thank the patient for his or her cooperation and use the alcohol gel at the end.

2.3 EXAMINATION OF THE NECK

Introduce yourself and gain consent for examining the patient's neck: 'Hello, I am Dr Jones. Would it be OK if I could examine your neck and swallowing?' Clean your hands with the alcohol gel.

Ask the patient if he or she currently has any pain in the neck.

Make sure the patient is sitting away from the wall, so you are able to fully examine the patient from behind.

Inspect the neck from all sides, making sure the patient's neck is adequately exposed to the clavicles.

Look for any obvious masses, scars or radiotherapy changes.

If there is an evidence of a thyroid mass/goitre then ask the patient to raise their hands above their head and look for facial plethora (Pemberton's sign – venous outflow obstruction in a narrowed thoracic inlet caused by an enlarged thyroid).

Ask the patient to stick out his or her tongue (assess for midline lumps that move with tongue protrusion, e.g. thyroglossal cyst).

Ask the patient to take a sip of water, hold it in his or her mouth and swallow on command. Assess for neck masses that move with swallowing (e.g. thyroid masses).

Assess the patient's voice by asking the patient to count to 10.

Begin palpating the neck from behind. Start midline over the trachea and assess that it is central. Move up the trachea over the larynx and level 6 nodes. Then palpate level 1 (submental and submandibular nodes), move down through levels 2, 3 and 4 and palpate supraclavicular and infraclavicular nodes. Work your way up the posterior body of the sternocleidomastoid in level 5 until you reach the occipital nodes. Palpate post- and pre-auricularly and, finally, palpate the parotid.

You do not need to follow this specific routine, but it is important to have a routine clear in your own mind that covers all regions of the neck (Figures 2.16–2.26).

Examine the parotid duct (opposite the upper second molar) and palpate the gland. It is also important to examine the facial nerve.

Thank the patient and close by using the alcohol gel.

In the examination there will not be any clinical signs to detect. However, for reference, any lump should be assessed for

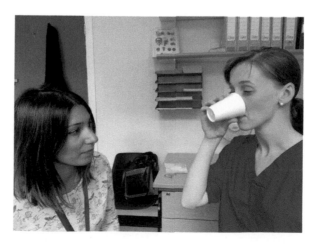

Figure 2.16 Swallow test.

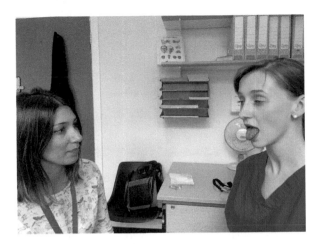

Figure 2.17 Tongue protrusion.

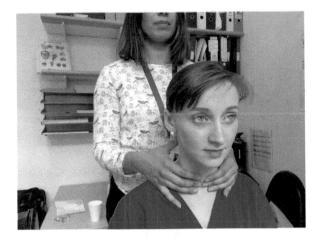

Figure 2.18 Examining the neck, palpating the trachea and level 6 nodes.

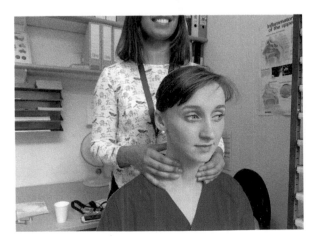

Figure 2.19 Checking the trachea is centralised.

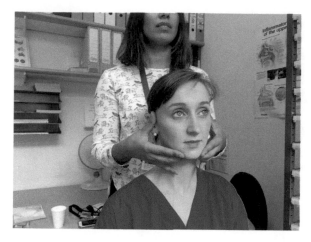

Figure 2.20 Palpation of level 1 nodes.

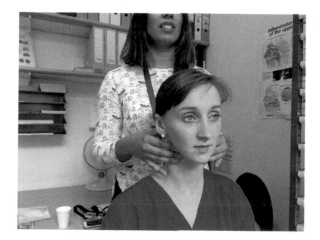

Figure 2.21 Palpation of level 2 nodes.

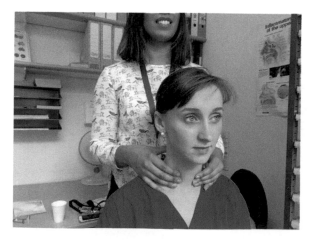

Figure 2.22 Palpation of levels 3 and 4 nodes.

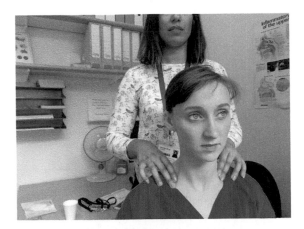

Figure 2.23 Palpation of supraclavicular nodes.

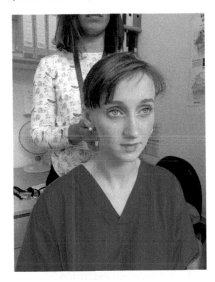

Figure 2.24 Palpation of occipital nodes.

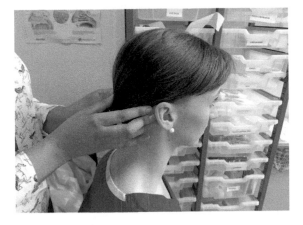

Figure 2.25 Palpation of occipital and post-auricular nodes.

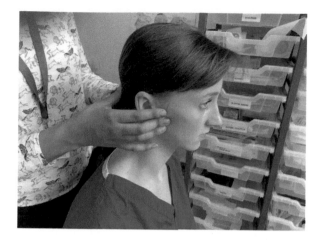

Figure 2.26 Palpation of the parotid.

- Site, size and surface
- Colour, contour and consistency
- Tenderness, temperature and transilluminability
- Pulsatility

If a mass is felt in the submandibular region, then attempt bimanual palpation of the gland through the floor of the mouth.

If a midline mass is felt, it is appropriate to take a thyroid history and examination.

On inspection, look for restlessness, sweating, vitiligo and clothing out of keeping with current climate.

Examine the patient's hands for tremor, sweating, palmar erythema, pretibial myxo-edema (Graves' dermopathy) and clubbing.

Move on to examining the eyes – check for lid lag and for loss of hair from the outer third of the eyebrows.

Check for chemosis and exophthalmos.

Percuss the upper sternum for retrosternal extension.

2.4   EXAMINATION OF THE ORAL CAVITY

Introduce yourself and gain consent for examining the patient's mouth: 'Hello, I am Dr Jones. Would it be OK if I could examine your mouth and throat?' Clean your hands with the alcohol gel.

Ask the patient if he or she currently has any pain. Ask the patient if he or she has dentures.

Ask the patient to open the mouth fully and say 'Ahh'. Perform a gross overview of the oral cavity. Assess any restriction in the mouth opening (Figure 2.27).

Using a tongue depressor, gently depress the tongue to inspect the soft palate, hard palate, uvula, tonsils and pillars (Figure 2.28).

Using two tongue blades, one in each hand, examine all teeth, gums and alveolar margins by lifting the lips away from the teeth. Start with the upper palate and then move to the lower palate (Figures 2.29–2.31).

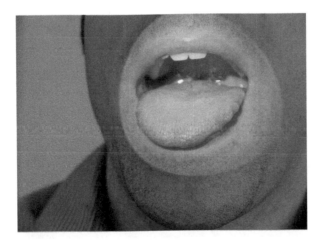

Figure 2.27 Examining the oral cavity, gross inspection.

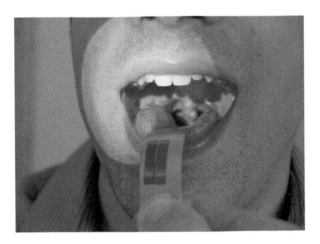

Figure 2.28 Use of Lack tongue depressor to examine soft palate, hard palate, uvula, tonsils and pillars.

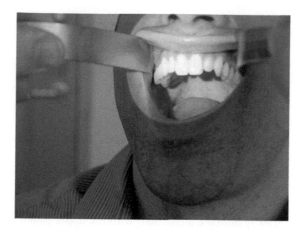

Figure 2.29 Use of Lack tongue depressor to examine upper teeth, gums and alveolar margins.

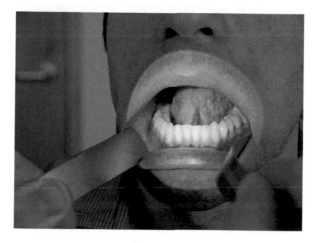

Figure 2.30 Use of Lack tongue depressor to examine lower teeth, gums and alveolar margins.

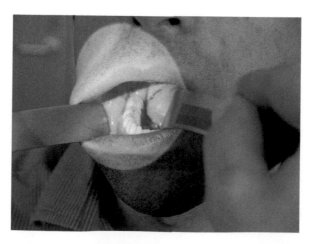

Figure 2.31 Use of Lack tongue depressor to examine the buccal membranes and parotid ducts.

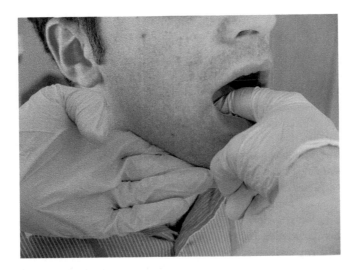

Figure 2.32 Bimanual palpation.

Use a blade to displace the tongue to one side and then the other side to examine the buccal membranes. Look opposite the second molars for the openings of the parotid ducts.

Ask the patient to lift the tongue up; inspect the floor of the mouth including the openings of the submandibular ducts.

If permitted by the examiner, proceed to put on a pair of disposable gloves and perform bimanual palpation of the following (Figure 2.32):

- Parotid gland and ducts
- Submandibular glands
- Floor of the mouth

Thank the patient and close by using the alcohol gel.

2.5 FLEXIBLE NASENDOSCOPY

This station typically involves an actor whom you talk to, while performing the actual nasendoscopy on a manikin. Many marks will be for communication skills – specifically, your ability to explain the procedure and reassure the patient throughout.

Always initiate the station by cleaning your hands with the alcohol gel.

Introduce yourself and gain consent for using a camera to look through the patient's nose and down at the voice box: 'Hi, I am Dr Jones. I would like to examine your voice box and nose with this flexible camera. Is that OK with you?'

Ask the patient if he or she currently has any pain.

Ask if the patient has ever had this procedure performed before.

Explain that you are using a thin camera called an endoscope that passes through the nose and points downwards into the throat so that the voice box can be examined. If there is a pen and paper provided, a diagram can be useful at this stage.

Reassure the patient that he or she may feel an awkward sensation during the procedure but that you can use a spray to numb the feeling and you can stop if it all becomes too uncomfortable.

Check with the patient if he or she has a preference for which nostril is to be used by asking if the patient breathes easier through a particular nostril or from any past experience with the procedure.

Explain you would spray the manikin's nostril with lidocaine/phenylephrine spray, asking the patient to simultaneously take a 'big sniff in'. Ideally you should wait 5 minutes. Explain to the examiner this is what you would do in the clinic; the examiner will usually tell you to continue.

Put on a pair of disposable gloves.

Take the endoscope and lubricate the end with jelly. Clean the lens with the alcohol wipe.

Slowly insert the endoscope into the chosen nostril of the manikin, reassuring the patient constantly that he or she is doing well. Hold the endoscope in your dominant hand while your non-dominant hand manoeuvres the end of the scope as it is enters the nostril.

Under vision through the scope, direct the scope towards the PNS, and then deflect the scope down towards the larynx (Figure 2.33).

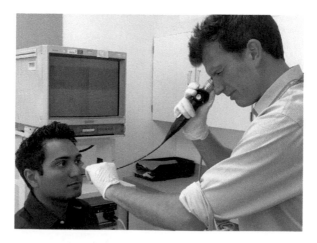

Figure 2.33 Flexible nasendoscopy.

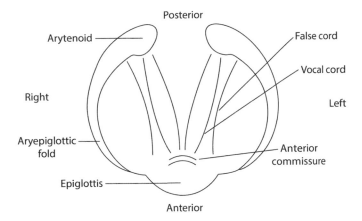

Figure 2.34 Diagram of the vocal tract as visualised by flexible nasendoscopy.

While visualising the larynx, ask the patient to perform three manoeuvres:

1. 'Say "Eee"'(to visualise adduction of vocal cords)
2. 'Stick your tongue out' (to visualise the valleculae)
3. 'Puff your cheeks out' (to visualise the piriform fossae)

Gently withdraw the scope, reassuring the patient.

Thank the patient and ensure the patient is comfortable again. Make sure you use the alcohol gel at the end.

You may be asked to draw your findings or make a drawing from a clinical photo. A schematic diagram of a normal larynx may look like **Figure** 2.34.

Often there is a picture with a vocal cord mass provided and you are asked to provide a labelled diagram. There are marks for labelling both the normal and the pathological areas. It is important that you can orientate (left, right, anterior, posterior) correctly from the photograph. This will come with practice. In the view shown in **Figure** 2.34, the left cord is on the right side of the diagram. Sometimes you are shown a picture taken under direct vision, using the rigid laryngoscope. Under direct vision, the cord of the left of the picture would be the left cord. The diagram in **Figure** 2.34, however, is an inverted view of the flexible nasendoscopy orientation that you are probably more used to.

2.6   VESTIBULAR ASSESSMENT

In recent years, the examination has included a balance station which may or may not include an ear examination. Therefore, it is important that you are just as slick in your vestibular assessment as you are in your ear exam to avoid getting flustered at this station.

Introduce yourself to the patient, explaining that you are going to be assessing the patient's balance: 'Hello, I am Dr Jones. I understand you've been having some trouble with your balance (or ears and balance). Would it be OK if I examined your balance today?'

Clean your hands with the alcohol gel provided before starting.

Tell the patient that you will be explaining what you're doing as you go along and let the patient know to ask if he or she has any questions. Ask if the patient is in any pain or discomfort. This is especially important for patients with osteoarthritis of their major joints or cervical spine as this may preclude parts of your examination, and you should show that you're aware of this.

WITH THE PATIENT SITTING

In the combined examination you should start with a thorough ear examination as described in a previous section unless specifically told to just examine the vestibular system.

Oculomotor testing

- Check for nystagmus (primary or gaze evoked)
- Ask the patient to keep the head still and follow your finger with his or her eyes completely in an H-shape (**Figure 2.35**).

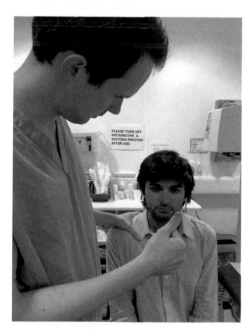

Figure 2.35 Assessing smooth pursuit.

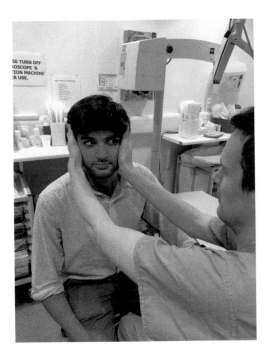

Figure 2.36 Vestibular–ocular reflex testing.

Test smooth pursuit and saccades

- Ask the patient to report any double vision or pain.
- State you would complete a full cranial nerve examination.

Cerebellar testing

- Dysdiadochokinesis and finger nose point for past-pointing
- Vestibular–ocular reflex (VOR)
  - Check for neck pain or reduced range of movement in the neck.
  - Tell the patient you will turn their head from side to side, asking him or her to focus on your nose.
  - Place your hands on the side of the head, avoid covering the ears (**Figure 2.36**).

In a normal head thrust test the eyes remain on the target.

WITH PATIENT STANDING

Romberg test

- Test of proprioceptive, vestibulo-spinal and cerebellar function.
- With the patient standing, feet together, hands by the sides, ask the patient to close his or her eyes and maintain that position.
- *Positive test* – Unable to maintain position in space, sways or falls during the test. Do not allow your patient to fall (**Figure 2.37**).

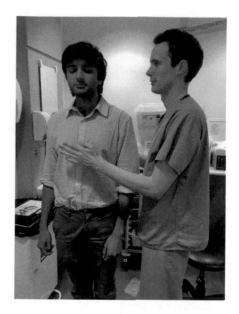

Figure 2.37 Romberg test.

Unterberger step test
Screening test for vestibular pathology.

- With the patient standing, ask the patient to stretch his or her arms out in front, palms up, eyes closed and marching on the spot.
- State you would do this for 60 seconds.
- Positive patient rotates on the spot towards the side that may have a labyrinthine lesion (**Figure 2.38**).

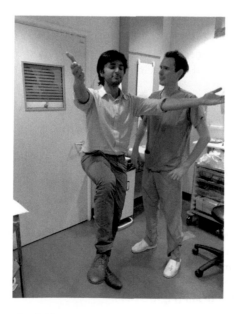

Figure 2.38 Unterberger step test.

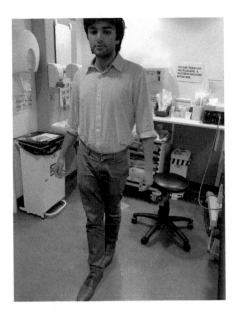

Figure 2.39 Heel–toe gait.

Heel–toe gait

- Test for general proprioceptive, pathway and coordination function.
- Ask the patient to walk in a straight line heel to toe and turn around and return to the start point (Figure 2.39).

WITH THE PATIENT ON THE COUCH

Dix–Hallpike test

- Test for benign paroxysmal positional vertigo (BPPV).
- Check for neck pain and restricted neck movement.
- Remember this test would be contraindicated in anyone with atlanto-axial instability, such as a patient with rheumatoid arthritis.
- Explain to the patient that you would like to test for the position of the crystals within the balance organ.
- Explain that this test may make him or her dizzy, but it shouldn't last for long.
- Position the patient sitting on the couch, legs extended. Rotate head 45 degrees to the test side. Lower the patient supporting the occiput, and extend the neck 20 degrees and hold in this position for 45 seconds observing the eyes for rotational nystagmus (beating towards the ground, geotropic) (Figure 2.40).

Positive test will have a fast phase of rotational nystagmus towards the affected ear (the test ear = the ear closer to the ground).

Following a positive test, confirming BPPV, you would proceed to perform the Epley manoeuvre having briefed the patient.

Thank the patient for his or her cooperation, state that you would now document your findings, and use the alcohol gel as you leave.

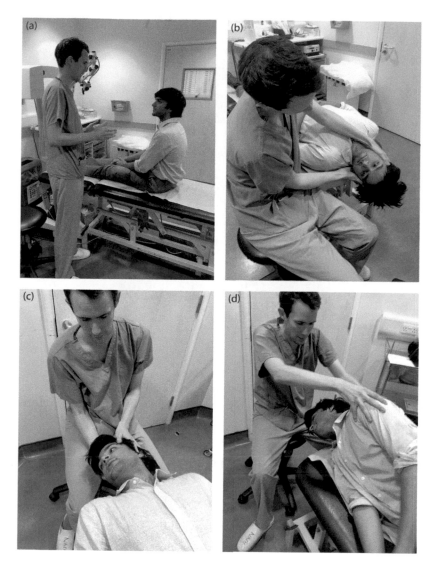

Figure 2.40 Dix–Hallpike testing.

Key features of nystagmus in the classic posterior canal BPPV are as follows:

- Latency of onset (5–10 seconds)
- Rotational geotropic nystagmus
- *Fatigable nystagmus* – Repeating the test with result in less nystagmus
- *Reversible* – Will eventually subside after a positive test upon sitting upright

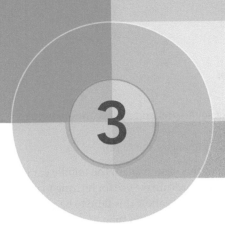

Communication Skills Stations

3.1 CONSENT STATIONS

Stations involving taking consent for operations feature prominently in the examination. It is important to remember that you are not required to take a history. The actors will be given some specific questions to ask the candidate. Make sure you answer these specifically, as they will certainly have marks awarded for the appropriate answer. The following are some example scenarios similar to those in the exam in previous years.

GROMMETS

Typical Scenario

You are the ENT junior doctor in a busy afternoon clinic with your consultant, Mr Powell. Your consultant has seen a 5-year-old girl with her mother. He has decided that the patient needs grommets for otitis media with effusion and has asked you to explain the procedure and take consent.

Time: 7 minutes

There will be a mother present; there will not be a child in the examination. Instead, the consultation is directed at informing the mother and answering her questions.

Introduce yourself and gauge the 'starting point'. It is important to find out what the mother has already been told and what she understands.

A useful question may be: 'I understand you have just spoken to the consultant, Mr Powell, and he feels that your daughter requires an operation. The operation he has suggested is the insertion of grommets into your daughter's eardrums. Do you understand what this entails?'

This will allow you to gauge the level of information that the patient requires to make an informed choice on whether to proceed with the operation.

Start by explaining the anatomy. A diagram can be helpful at this stage. There are often 'props' available such as a model of an ear. Marks are awarded for their use, so make sure you use them if they are provided.

Explain that the ear is divided into three sections:

1. The outer ear (the part you can see)
2. The middle ear (where the bones that conduct sound are) and a tube (the eustachian tube) that connects to the nose
3. The inner ear (where sound is made into nerve signals for the brain)

Explain the reasons for performing the operation. In this case, explain the middle ear has filled with thick fluid, or 'glue', that is not allowing the eardrum we use for hearing to move properly. Explain that we will make a hole in the eardrum to allow this fluid to be removed by suction during the operation. We then put in a small ventilation tube (it can be helpful to draw one if one is not provided) that prevents further fluid accumulation by ventilating the middle ear. This should help the eardrum move more easily with sound and should also help the child to hear more easily.

The grommets will stay in the ear for an average of 6–9 months. They tend to fall out naturally and do not need to be removed.

On the basis of the appearance of the eardrum, the child's reduced hearing (at home and on the audiogram test) and the pressure tests, it is recommended that we proceed with placing the grommets.

Explain the alternatives to surgery. In this case, explain that it is true that most children will grow out of this problem but, unfortunately, this is a very important point in their development. Children may suffer from speech and language delay and/or behavioural problems if we do not treat them. In cases where grommets are not appropriate or not desired hearing aids may be offered.

Explain the procedure. In this case, explain that it is a quick operation (approximately 10 minutes) that requires a short general anaesthetic (explain they will be seen by the anaesthetist later, and the anaesthetist will be able to answer any of their questions regarding this).

Explain what will happen after the operation. In this case, explain that it is advisable to keep the ears dry when washing for the first few days after the operation.

The mother may specifically ask about swimming. Advise her that this is usually permissible but that some patients may prefer to use a headband or earplugs. Diving is never advised. Explain they will be seen in clinic in about 3 months to check progress.

Explain the risks of surgery. In this case, explain that it is a safe operation but the patient should be aware of the risks, as with any surgery.

- *Infection* – This is rare but is usually easily manageable with antibiotic ear drops.
- *A persistent perforation (hole in the eardrum)* – Sometimes this needs another operation.
- There may be a small amount of pain or bleeding, but this usually settles very quickly.

If a consent form is provided, then it should be filled in with the parent. Offer to give a copy of the consent form to the patient. It is not usual that a consent form will be provided in the examination.

Ask if they have any questions. Make sure the parent has follow-up information, e.g. the clinic or ward phone number in case of concerns (Table 3.1).

Table 3.1 Example Mark Scheme

	Yes	No	Outstanding
Shows environment considerations (e.g. suitable seating arrangement)			
Makes introduction			
Establishes rapport			
Uses appropriate non-verbal communication			
Establishes patient's understanding			
Establishes patient's level of information requirement			
Shows professionalism			
Uses appropriate terminology			
Outlines procedure			
Explains indications			
Explains important complications			
Gives information in manageable amounts			
Checks understanding			
Summarises			
Closes appropriately			
Offers follow-up, extra sources of information			

FUNCTIONAL ENDOSCOPIC SINUS SURGERY

Typical Scenario

A 55-year-old man has been troubled by recurrent sinusitis for the last 10 years. Your consultant has seen the patient and has decided to perform functional endoscopic sinus surgery (FESS). The consultant has asked you to explain the procedure and to take informed consent.

Time: 7 minutes

Start by gauging the patient's starting point with a general opening statement such as: 'Perhaps you could bring me up to speed about what you've already been told about the operation'. From this you can gauge how much background information you will need to give to the patient.

Explain the anatomy of the sinuses: 'The sinuses are air- and mucus-filled spaces in the bones of the face and head. Sinusitis is an infection of these spaces. This is what has been giving you the symptoms of nasal obstruction and nasal discharge. Topical nasal steroids and antibiotics treat most sinusitis. However, in severe cases like yours this has not been able to treat it satisfactorily and an operation is required to open up the sinuses to allow the medication to take effect'.

Explain the reasons for performing the surgery: '"Functional endoscopic sinus surgery" is sinus surgery undertaken using a telescopic camera or "endoscope". This means we do not need to make any cuts to the outside of the face and we can do the whole operation via the nose. We will be aiming to open up the drainage pathways. This will help the flow of mucus and will stop the sinuses becoming inflamed and infected. This is normally an effective procedure, although, sometimes it has to be done more than once. Once the sinuses have been opened medication will more easily access the inflamed sinus linings so it is very important that you continue to use the prescribed topical nasal steroids after the operation'.

Explain the alternatives to surgery: 'It would be possible to continue to have nasal steroid drops, courses of antibiotics and occasional courses of oral steroids, but these will not combat severe cases. There is also a risk of serious eye and brain infections spreading from infected sinuses'.

Explain the procedure: 'You will require a general anaesthetic (explain the anaesthetist will answer any questions about the anaesthetic). The operation is done inside the nose without any cuts to the face. The operation usually lasts 45 minutes. After the operation you may have some nasal packing for the first 24 hours. It is common to have a blocked nose and some bloody nasal discharge for a few days after the operation'.

Explain what will happen after the operation: 'You will be able to go home on the same day usually. It is important not to blow your nose for the first 48 hours after the operation. Some surgeons also advise nasal douching, which means irrigating the nose with salty water, usually starting on postoperative day 3. You will need to continue using the nasal steroid sprays. You will be given instructions about this before you leave the ward'.

Explain it is routine to have 1 week off work and 2 weeks off strenuous exercise. Explain the risks of surgery. In this case, explain that although this operation is performed regularly without any problems there are some serious risks of which the patient should be aware:

- *Bleeding* – It is very common to have some small quantity of bleeding from the nose and to have blood-tinged mucus for a few days after the operation.
- *Bleeding into the eye* – This is rare but can cause black eyes that will recover on their own. A more serious bleed into the eye can result if there is damage to a main artery. Although this is very rare, there is a chance that you could lose the sight in the eye. If this does happen, you may need another operation. In a recent audit in the United Kingdom, eye complications happened in 1 in 500 operations.
- *Cerebrospinal fluid (CSF) leak* – The sinuses lie right under the base of the brain, which is contained in special fluid called CSF. A small leak can occur via the nose if there is some bony damage. This often requires no treatment and will recover on its own. Occasionally, you may need another operation to seal over the leak. Sometimes an infection can get into the fluid that will require the use of antibiotics. CSF leaks occur in about 1 in 1000 operations.

If available, fill in the consent form with the patient. Offer to give a copy of the consent form to the patient.

Ask if the patient has any questions. Make sure the patient has follow-up information, e.g. the clinic or ward phone number in case of concerns.

SEPTOPLASTY

Typical Scenario

You are asked to see a patient on the ward who has been admitted electively for a septoplasty. Explain the procedure to the patient and take informed consent.

Time: 7 minutes

First off, ascertain the patient's understanding of the operation with a general open question such as: 'Can you tell me how much you have been told about the operation?'

Explain the reason for performing the operation: 'The septum is a piece of cartilage inside the nose separating the left and right nostrils. In most people the septum is not straight; however, in some people this can cause a blocked nose on one side. This operation is done to try to straighten the septum and to improve the airflow through the nose'.

Explain the alternatives to surgery: 'The operation is only undertaken when symptoms are very troubling. No harm will result from not undertaking the procedure'.

Explain the procedure: 'The operation is done through the nose and there are no cuts to the outside of the face. You shouldn't get any bruising to the face. The operation is done under general anaesthesia and you will be seen by an anaesthetist who can answer any questions about the anaesthetic. The operation takes about 45 minutes'.

Explain what will happen after the operation: 'Sometimes you will have some nasal packing, which needs to be kept in overnight. You can normally go home on the same day. You will need 1 week off work and 2 weeks off strenuous exercise'. Explain the risks of the operation: 'Septal surgery is safe surgery; however, there are some complications of which you need to be aware':

- *Bleeding* – We may place 'packs' into the nose, overnight to absorb any bleeding. These will be removed before you leave the ward.

  It is very common to get some bloody discharge from the nose for the first couple of weeks. Larger bleeds can happen, most commonly within the first 2 weeks. On very rare occasions you might need to return to the operating theatre to stop a large bleed. There is also a chance of a blood clot or 'haematoma' forming around the wound. If this happens it is very likely that you would need to go back to theatre to have it treated.
- *Pain* – This is usually manageable with painkillers.
- *Continued blocked nose* – It will take at least 2 weeks for the nose to start feeling 'normal' again. However, we cannot guarantee alleviation of your symptoms.
- *Change to appearance of the nose* – As the septum provides support to the structure of the nose, there is a chance that the appearance of the nose can change. This is very unlikely if this is your first operation; however, with repeat operations the chances increase. In serious cases the nose can collapse.
- *Septal perforation* – There is a chance that a hole can form in the septum, causing a connection between the left and right nostrils. This often causes minimal problems such as bleeding and crusting and requires no further treatment. Ongoing perforations may need another operation to repair.

Numbness of the top teeth which are close to the floor of the nose is an occasional risk.

If available, fill in the consent form with the patient. Offer to give a copy of the consent form to the patient.

Ask if the patient has any questions. Make sure the patient has follow-up information, e.g. the clinic or ward phone number in case of concerns.

PANENDOSCOPY AND MICROLARYNGOSCOPY

Typical Scenario

A 65-year-old man has had a hoarse voice for the last 6 weeks. He is due to have a microlaryngoscopy and biopsy. Explain the procedure to him and take consent.

Time: 7 minutes

First off, ascertain the patient's starting point with a general open question such as: 'Can you tell me how much you have been told about the operation?'

Explain the reason for performing the procedure: 'We need to have a look at the voice box and the throat. We have probably already looked at the voice box in the clinic but now we need to have a better look under a general anaesthetic. Sometimes we need to take a section of tissue so it can be examined in the pathology laboratory'.

Explain the alternatives to surgery: 'Unfortunately, if we are to best manage this condition we need to see the voice box directly by undertaking this procedure'. Explain the procedure: 'The consultant will use a metal tube (laryngoscope and oesophagoscope) and a microscope to visualise the voice box. We will also be able to examine your nose, mouth and the rest of your throat at this time. The procedure lasts about 15 minutes'.

Explain what will happen after the procedure: 'Most patients have a sore throat after the procedure. This is usually manageable with painkillers. Some surgeons ask that you rest your voice for 24–48 hours if a biopsy has been performed. Some patients have a sore neck from the position during the operation. This usually settles without any treatment, but you should inform us if you have any long-standing neck problems. You can usually go home the same day. You will be able to eat and drink as you are able after the operation, unless the surgeon instructs differently'.

Explain the risks of the procedure:

Injury to lining of the throat – The risks are small but you should be aware that there is a risk of scratching the lining of the throat. This can cause some blood to come up in your saliva. If we take some tissue for a biopsy, the chances of bleeding are raised. Normally bleeding is easy to deal with during the operation, rarely there is significant bleeding in the airway. This would be an emergency and may require a tracheostomy (breathing tube through the neck) as a life saving procedure.

When we are looking further down the throat (oesophagoscopy), if the damage is more severe, such as a perforation or hole in the gullet, there is a chance that you would need to stay in hospital and receive feeding through a tube through the nose until the injury has healed. It is also possible that you would need an operation to repair the perforation.

Damage to teeth – There is a small risk that we can chip some teeth when we put in the metal tube. Often we use a gum guard to protect the teeth. If any damage is done we will arrange to repair the teeth at a later date.

Explain that you will see them in clinic with results.

If available, fill in the consent form with the patient. Offer to give a copy of the consent form to the patient.

Ask if the patient has any questions. Make sure the patient has follow-up information, e.g. the clinic or ward phone number in case of concerns.

MYRINGOPLASTY

Typical Scenario

A 24-year-old man has a long-standing dry perforation of his right eardrum. The consultant has decided to perform a myringoplasty. Explain the procedure to the patient and take consent.

Time: 7 minutes

Start by gauging the patient's starting point.

Explain the anatomy of the ear. The use of a quick diagram here can be very useful to describe the three sections of the ear:

1. The outer ear (the part you can see)

2. The middle ear (where the bones that conduct sound are) and a tube (the eustachian tube) that connects to the nose
3. The inner ear (where sound is made into nerve signals for the brain)

The eardrum connects the outer ear to the middle ear.

Explain the reasons for the operation: 'Most perforations are self-healing, but ones that do not heal often need an operation. The aim is to reduce the number of infections you are getting by sealing the middle ear from the outer ear. Some people notice an improvement in their hearing but we cannot guarantee this'.

Explain the alternatives to surgery: 'Without an operation the ear may continue to get infected. With this operation we hope to cut down the risk of ear infections'.

Explain the procedure: 'Often it is possible to perform the operation down the ear canal but sometimes a cut is made behind the ear or above the ear canal in the crease of skin. A small piece of cartilage is often taken from the tragus or conchal bowl (demonstrate these to the patient). This tissue is used to repair the hole as a graft. If there is a skin incision it is then stitched closed and a head bandage is applied'.

Explain the risks of the operation: 'The operation has a high success rate, although it is lower if the hole is large or if you are having a lot of infections':

- Failure of the operation to repair the hole in 10%–15% of cases. This may mean a further operation is required.
- *Hearing loss* – There is a small risk that the hearing can decrease or even be completely lost on the operated side.
- *Taste disturbance* – The nerve that supplies taste to the tongue runs under the eardrum. Damage to this nerve can result in some abnormal taste on one side of the tongue. People often describe it as a metallic taste. This is usually temporary, although it can be a permanent change.
- *Ringing in the ear or tinnitus* – This can be temporary or permanent.
- There is a small risk that the wound can become infected; if so, this may need treatment with antibiotics.
- *Dizziness* – This is common for a few hours following surgery. On rare occasions, dizziness is prolonged.
- *Facial paralysis* – The nerve that supplies the muscles that move the face runs very close to the eardrum. Any damage to this nerve can cause a paralysis of the face; however, this is exceedingly rare in this operation. Recovery can be complete or partial.

If available, fill in the consent form with the patient. Offer to give a copy of the consent form to the patient.

Ask if the patient has any questions. Make sure the patient has follow-up information, e.g. the clinic or ward phone number in case of concerns.

PAROTID SURGERY

Typical Scenario

A 76-year-old man has had a unilateral swelling over his parotid gland for the last year. It has steadily increased in size. Fine needle aspiration and ultrasound have been performed that are suggestive of pleomorphic adenoma. He has been listed for a right-sided superficial parotidec-tomy. Explain the procedure and take consent.

Time: 7 minutes

Start by gauging the patient's starting point.

Explain the anatomy and function of the parotid glands: 'The parotid glands are paired salivary glands on the side of the face, running from behind the ears to lie over the jaw'. (A diagram may be helpful at this stage.)

Explain the reasons for the operation: 'Parotid lumps are usually benign and not cancerous. In your case, the first tests have suggested that it is not a cancer but these lumps will carry on growing. They can begin to look very large and there is a small chance that they can become cancerous, so we like to operate on them as soon as possible. The only way of being certain of the diagnosis is to remove the lump and send it to the laboratory'.

Explain the alternatives to surgery: 'Because of the risks previously mentioned, we like to remove this type of parotid lump; therefore, there is no alternative treatment available other than to do nothing'.

Explain the procedure: 'The operation is performed under general anaesthesia. You will see an anaesthetist who can answer any questions about the anaesthetic. The operation is done through a cut in front of the ear and down into the neck. In most people the scar heals very well'.

Explain what will happen after the operation: 'Most surgeons will insert a small drain into the neck for the first 24 hours to make sure no blood can collect in the wound. You can usually go home 48 hours after the operation or once the drain is removed and the surgeon is happy with your progress. It is advised that you take 2 weeks off work'.

Explain the risks of surgery: 'Parotid surgery is generally safe, but there are some risks that you should be aware of':

- *Facial weakness* – The most serious risk is damage to the nerve that moves the facial muscles. The nerve is very closely intertwined with the gland and, although great care is taken to protect the nerve, in about 20% of people there is some weakness of the face on the operated side. In most cases this is temporary, although in about 1% of cases there is a permanent weakness.
- *Numbness of the face and ear* – There is some numbness to the side of the face in the majority of people and this usually recovers in time. However, often the nerve that supplies sensation to the earlobe is cut and the earlobe will be permanently numb.
- *Haematoma or blood clot* – Bleeding under the skin can happen in about 5% of people. Occasionally this blood clot can become infected. Rarely, people need to go back to theatre to stop this bleed.
- *Salivary collection* – In about 5% of people there can be leaking of saliva under the skin from the remaining parotid gland. This can collect in the first few weeks after surgery and needs to be drained with a needle. Usually no other treatment is required.
- *Frey's syndrome* – Some patients find that after this surgery their cheek can become hot and sweaty while eating. This is because a nerve has grown back slightly in the wrong place. Often this will settle down with time and requires no further treatment. If symptoms are more troublesome then antiperspirant or Botox can be used.

If available, fill in the consent form with the patient. Offer to give a copy of the consent form to the patient.

Ask if the patient has any questions. Make sure the patient has follow-up information, e.g. the clinic or ward phone number in case of concerns.

SUBMANDIBULAR SURGERY

Typical Scenario

A 46-year-old female is having recurrent infections of a submandibular gland secondary to a salivary gland calculus, and has been placed on the list for a removal of the gland. Explain the procedure to her and take consent.

Time: 7 minutes

Start by gauging the patient's starting point.

Explain the anatomy: 'The submandibular glands are two salivary glands underneath the jaw. They produce saliva when we eat. Because the saliva can be quite thick there is a chance that stones can form. These can cause infections. The aim of this operation is to remove one of the glands to stop these infections. Your ability to eat should not be affected, as there are a number of other salivary glands that can still produce saliva'.

Explain the reasons for the operation: 'In your case the duct is not draining efficiently, as it is blocked with a stone. This is causing the infections and pain'.

Explain the alternatives to surgery: 'Infections can be treated with antibiotics but an operation is needed to remove the stone'.

Explain the procedure: 'The operation is undertaken with a general anaesthetic. A cut is made under the jaw and the gland is removed'.

Explain what will happen after the operation: 'A drain will be placed into the wound for the first 24 hours after the operation. You can usually go home the next day. You will need 1 week off work'.

Explain the risks of the operation:

- Haematoma or blood clot can form under the skin in about 5% of people. This may require a return to the operating theatre to stop the bleed.
- *Infection* – Uncommonly the wound can become infected. This is because there was infection in the gland. Sometimes pus will need to be drained from the wound and antibiotics started.
- *Facial weakness* – The nerve that makes the lower lip move runs very close to the gland. This is called the marginal mandibular branch of the facial nerve. If this is damaged it can cause a drooping of the lower lip. This can be temporary or permanent.
- There is a chance that the area of skin around the wound will be numb. This usually improves with time but there can be permanent changes.
- *Numbness of tongue and changes in taste* – The nerve that supplies sensation and taste to the operated side of the tongue runs very close to the gland. Damage will cause changes that can be temporary or permanent.
- Injury to the nerve that 'moves' the tongue. The nerve that moves the tongue runs close to the gland. Damage to this nerve is very uncommon.

If available, fill in the consent form with the patient. Offer to give a copy of the consent form to the patient.

Ask if the patient has any questions. Make sure the patient has follow-up information, e.g. the clinic or ward phone number in case of concerns.

3.2   EXPLANATION STATIONS

These stations ask you to explain an ENT diagnosis to a patient or relative. You are given time to prepare with the information for the scenario provided on the rest station before so have plenty of time to read, re-read and plan your structured approach. You may also be provided paper that can be used to prepare simple diagrams to aid your explanation.

BENIGN PAROXYSMAL POSITIONAL VERTIGO

Typical Scenario

A 48-year-old man has a new diagnosis of benign paroxysmal positional vertigo (BPPV). Please explain the diagnosis and answer his questions.

Time: 7 minutes

Introduce yourself and confirm you are talking to the correct patient.

Start with an open question such as: 'I understand you have a new diagnosis of benign paroxysmal positional vertigo. I was wondering if you could tell me what you've been told about it'. This will give you the opportunity to explore the patient's current knowledge and obviously the subsequent explanation will be tailored to this.

It is useful to get a summary history from the patient as to the symptoms he or she is having and the time course of onset (e.g. post-traumatic BPPV occurs after head injury as opposed to the more insidious onset of idiopathic BPPV). However, the history is not the focus of this station and so you should not waste much time on history taking, as there will not be many marks on offer.

There will be marks available for exploring the ideas, concerns and expectations of the patient. It may be useful to ask if the patient has known anyone else with this condition. There may be underlying worries, e.g. a relative with vertigo who subsequently was diagnosed with a central nervous system tumour.

Move on to the explanation of the pathology. This will be aided by the use of diagrams of the ear and semicircular canals.

Explain the ear consists of outer, middle and inner divisions and this problem involves the inner ear.

Explain that the inner ear senses balance by the position of calcium crystals. In the patient's case, some of the crystals have moved from where they should be (utricle) to one of the canals. Hence, when the patient moves his or her head the fluid shifts and causes the vertigo.

Explain the treatment is to move the head in a certain manner to realign the crystals (the Epley procedure). Explain this is an extremely effective procedure in most patients.

If the patient is still having problems, the procedure can be repeated. There are also vestibular rehabilitation exercises. You can offer to give the patient a leaflet detailing these.

Explain surgery is rarely required but is the last resort. This can involve blocking one of the semicircular canals (posterior) or cutting the balance nerves or destroying the vestibular system.

Ask if the patient has any further questions. Ensure that there are follow-up procedures in place (Table 3.2).

Table 3.2 Example Mark Scheme

	Yes	No	Outstanding
Shows environmental considerations (e.g. suitable seating arrangement)			
Makes introduction			
Establishes rapport			
Uses appropriate non-verbal communication			
Establishes patient's understanding			
Establishes patient's level of information requirement			
Shows professionalism			
Asks suitable opening question			
Listens to patient's history			
Facilitates appropriately			
Summarises information and asks for clarification			
Establishes hidden agenda			
Is succinct/relevant			

CHOLESTEATOMA

Typical Scenario

A 12-year-old child presents to the outpatient clinic with a history of right-sided hearing loss and chronic otorrhoea. The consultant has previously seen the patient and diagnosed cholesteatoma, requiring surgery in the form of a mastoidectomy. Explain the diagnosis, further investigations and the procedure to the mother.

Time: 7 minutes

First, introduce yourself as you would in a normal clinical scenario, stating your name and confirming the patient's identity.

Start by gauging the parent's understanding of the diagnosis and further management with an open question such as: 'Can you tell me what has happened so far and how much you have been told about the diagnosis?'

At this point the parent will know the diagnosis and have specific concerns relating to this, or if diagnosis has not been broached before, then the next part of the consultation takes similar structure to a breaking bad news station.

Either way it is often useful to recap the presenting complaint, hearing test results and examination findings. This acts to set the scene for delivering the diagnosis and discussing further management.

Reviewing the hearing test (usually available) will typically show unilateral conductive hearing loss.

Explain the findings on examination using diagrams to help you explain the structure of the ear in terms of outer canal, middle bones of hearing and inner organs of hearing and balance. You could explain the findings on examination in simple terms as a collection of skin cells in the wrong place.

This collection of skin cells is called cholesteatoma, and this is the cause of the symptoms he has been having.

Reassurance will be needed at this point to emphasise that this is not a tumour/cancer or cholesterol problem.

Explain the pathology in simple terms such as a collection of skin cells in the wrong place that can become infected causing discharge and hearing loss through damage to the bones of hearing.

At this point the parent may have specific questions he or she wishes to ask, and it would be a good time to explore the parent's ideas, concerns and expectations.

The parent may have concerns about permanent hearing loss, and some reassurance about the nature of the hearing loss will be required, emphasising the possibility for good hearing outcomes if justified by the pure-tone audiometry (PTA) provided, leading into the discussion of further management. Hearing outcomes will depend upon the severity and nature of the loss (conductive hearing loss [CHL]/sensorineural hearing loss [SNHL]/mixed).

Again an open question about the patient's understanding of the treatments for this condition would be appropriate.

Explain the further investigations that are required. Computed tomography (CT) of temporal bones is conducted to look for the extent of local damage and to help plan for surgery.

Introduce the otology multidisciplinary team (MDT) and the members who will be involved in the decision making with the involvement of the parent, but the mainstay of treatment is surgery with an operation called a mastoidectomy.

Explain the procedure in terms of intended benefit, dependent on disease extent. Mastoidectomy is an operation usually performed with an incision behind the ear, to establish the extent of disease and clear all of the skin cells. The bones of hearing may or may not need to be addressed. If they do, this can be done at the time or as a second-stage procedure. Any holes in or retracted areas of the ear drum can also be addressed.

It is important to explain the potential consequences of not treating, with further hearing loss, progressing to damage to the organs of hearing and balance and eventually a dead ear, tinnitus, risk of recurrent infection, including spread of infection to the brain, injury to the facial nerve causing facial weakness.

These are also the risks of surgery, in addition to pain and bleeding. However, surgery is performed in a controlled manner and aims to clear disease, halting the destructive process and these risks are small, whereas we know that, if left unchecked, the cholesteatoma will lead to significant morbidity for the patient.

Ask if they have any further questions and make sure they have further follow-up arranged and contact details for the secretaries if they need to contact the team. Give them a patient information leaflet for further reading.

Thank the parent and close.

THY3F THYROID NODULE

Typical Scenario

A 35-year-old woman has returned to your outpatient clinic after fine needle aspiration (FNA) of a thyroid nodule. The cytology has been reported as Thy3F. Please explain the results, discuss further management and answer any questions.

Time: 7 minutes

Start by introducing yourself, stating your name and grade and confirming the patient's identity.

You should begin with an open question to recap what has happened so far and gauge the patient's understanding such as, 'Can you tell me in your own words what has happened so far and what you have been told about this?'

Then a summary history of the presentation is a useful recap; this will often be an asymptomatic midline neck lump picked up on examination or incidentally on CT/magnetic resonance imaging (MRI)/ultrasound of the neck for another indication. This is not the focus of the station so should only be a brief recap to avoid running out of time.

It is important to remember the patients 'hidden agenda', and this can be explored here by enquiring about the patient's ideas, concerns and expectations. In a station like this the patient may be a professional voice user and have specific concerns regarding surgery and the risks of a hoarse voice, for example.

Recapping the indication for the ultrasound-guided fine needle aspiration cytology is a useful way of leading into discussing the result and further management. At this time you can refer to your prepared diagram showing the thyroid's position in the neck, saying something such as 'we take a needle sample of tissue from the lump and examine this in the lab to try to differentiate a benign from cancerous lump'.

The same is graded according to the appearances of the cells and the likelihood of them being cancerous.

In the case of Thy3F nodules we cannot make this distinction on cytology alone and approximately one third of these nodules will be cancerous. Current practice would then be to proceed to diagnostic hemithyroidectomy for an accurate diagnosis and inform the MDT to enable decision making for further management as indicated.

Having explained this result to the patient, it is important to check the patient's understanding.

It is important to emphasise that at this point we are unable to say whether or not the lump is benign without removing more tissue and having a closer look under the microscope. If it is benign, then no further treatment will be required, and if not, then we will be able to discuss what further treatment is needed. There won't be the time or the need to go into this during this station.

Again check the patient's understanding so far, answering specific questions.

Explain the procedure. This should be done while referring to the diagram. Performed under general anaesthetic, it usually takes 90 minutes. While referring to the diagram, explain the position of the horizontal cut in the neck that will leave a thin scar.

Explain what will happen after the operation: 'This operation usually doesn't require a drain and you typically go home the same day, but sometimes you stay overnight and go home the next day. You will need 1 week off work'.

Explain the risks of the operation:

- *Haematoma or blood clot* – This can form under the skin and may require return to theatre to stop the bleeding.
- *Infection* – Uncommonly the wound can become infected. This would require antibiotics and, if a collection of infection forms, then may require another procedure to wash out the infection, but this is uncommon.
- *Hoarse voice* – This can occur if the nerve, called the recurrent laryngeal nerve, is irritated or stretched during the operation. If damaged, this can lead to hoarse voice that can be temporary or permanent. This is uncommon, and we use a nerve monitor to alert to any irritation during the procedure.

We only remove half of the thyroid gland, so at this point it will not impact the function of the gland and you will not need to take any hormone replacement pills. In a minority of patients the remaining half of the thyroid stops working so we recommend thyroid function tests 3 months after the operation.

Check understanding, offer opportunity to ask questions, provide patient information and ensure the patient has the contact details for the department should he or she want to get in touch.

Thank the patient and close.

VESTIBULAR SCHWANNOMA

Typical Scenario

A 45-year-old woman returns to your outpatient clinic for review after MRI internal auditory meatus (IAM) was performed to investigate moderate left-sided SNHL. The MRI shows a 2.2 cm vestibular schwannoma at the left cerebellopontine angle. Discuss the diagnosis and explain the further management.

Time: 7 minutes

First, introduce yourself as you would in a normal clinical scenario, stating your name and confirming the patient's identity.

Start by gauging the parent's understanding of the diagnosis and further management with an open question such as: 'Can you tell me what has happened so far and how much you have been told about the diagnosis?'

A summary history of the presentation is a useful recap and informs you of the current problems. This will often include unilateral SNHL but not always. If a PTA is available, this should be reviewed at this time.

The patient will have had an MRI of the internal acoustic meatus and will be returning for the results. Before discussing the scan results you can explore the patient's ideas, concerns and expectations.

Then frame this section by recapping the reason for doing the investigation: 'to look at the organs of hearing and balance and the nerve supplying them to exclude a swelling on the nerve that could be causing your symptoms'.

Then provide the warning shot as you would do in a breaking bad news station, 'unfortunately I have some bad news' or 'I am afraid our suspicions were confirmed'.

Explanation of the pathology: Using the scan if provided, or a simple diagram, explain the structure of the ear in terms of outer canal, middle bones of hearing and inner organs of hearing and balance supplied by nerves from the brain.

A vestibular schwannoma is a swelling of the nerve of balance that causes problems because it presses on nerves next to it – nerve of hearing, facial nerve, nerve for facial sensation – and relate this to the problems they have presented with.

It is important to emphasise that this isn't a cancer, which will often be a concern that needs addressing.

Vestibular schwannoma are uncommon and the majority do not grow. In some people they do grow but they tend to grow very slowly (1–2 mm/year). It has likely the tumour has been there for many years only presenting now as it has reached a certain size.

At this point check the understanding and address any questions.

Explain the treatment options. Introduce the Neurotology MDT composed of specialists who will discuss the best treatment plan and make a decision with you.

Treatment options include

- Watch and wait with surveillance scanning (MRI)
- Radiotherapy (gamma knife stereotactic radiosurgery)
- Surgery (hearing preserving and non-preserving techniques)

Addressing return of hearing after surgery – Explain that return of hearing will be variable and depend on size of the vestibular schwannoma, current level of hearing and treatment. There are options to address hearing after surgery and they can be discussed in more detail after the MDT discussion. Keep things as simple as possible as time will be limited.

Check the understanding, offer opportunity to ask questions and provide patient information. Ensure follow-up is booked for after the Neurotology MDT and the contact details for the department are given, should the patient want to get in touch.

Thank the patient and close.

3.3   BREAKING BAD NEWS

These can be potentially very difficult stations, with a number of unpredictable variables. It is important to remain calm and composed throughout the scenario, as it is easy to become flustered by outward shows of emotion from the actor, even in the artificial setting of an examination.

Typical Scenario

Mr Jones is a 48-year-old man who has been given a diagnosis of supraglottic laryngeal cancer at his last consultant appointment. He has returned to clinic today with some questions.

Time: 7 minutes

Introduce yourself and make sure you are addressing the correct patient.

Place yourself in a non-threatening position, e.g. no barriers such as desks between you and the patient.

Ask if the patient has brought anyone with him. You can offer to bring in a nurse if he would find that helpful.

Start with an open question to gauge the starting position of the patient: 'Mr Jones, perhaps you could just bring me up to speed as to what you have been told so far'. This will guide the whole scenario. It is important to establish the patient's agenda: 'Perhaps you could give me a list of questions that you would like me to answer and I will do my best to advise you'.

Often, as in real clinic scenarios, patients cannot remember very much after hearing bad news, so it is very likely in this situation that you will need to take the explanation from the beginning.

Explain the diagnosis – always start with a 'warning shot' to prepare the patient for the news. Something like: 'I am sorry, but the news is not what we wanted to hear'. Proceed then with a clear explanation of the condition, explaining any difficult terms. A diagram is very useful here. The patient may react in a number of ways (anger, crying, bargaining). Try to remain supportive but composed. If physical contact such as a hand on the shoulder seems appropriate to you, then this can be a useful strategy to improve rapport. Always give the patient plenty of time to react (you do not need to say anything but, rather, use your body language to facilitate the patient's reaction; this is a useful tactic for uncovering the patient's primary concerns).

There will often be extra marks for revealing underlying concerns, e.g. 'Who will take care of my children?' These can be teased out with questions like: 'I know this is a real shock, but is there anything else that you're worried about?'

Try to remain positive, but do not be falsely reassuring. For example, in this instance explain there are a number of treatment options open (radiotherapy, surgery, etc.).

If the patient wants to address causative factors ('Am I to blame, doctor? Was it the smoking?'), you must allow the patient to do this without interjecting value-laden statements. For example, here it is correct to say: 'Smoking is a known risk factor for this disease, but we can never be certain that this is the only cause'. It can be helpful at this stage to stress the treatment options.

Summarise the information you have given the patient and check that the patient understands.

Table 3.3 Example Mark Scheme

	Yes	No	Outstanding
Shows environmental considerations (e.g. suitable seating arrangement)			
Makes introduction			
Establishes rapport			
Uses appropriate non-verbal communication			
Establishes patient's understanding			
Establishes patient's level of information requirement			
Shows professionalism			
Ascertains if patient is accompanied			
Invites relatives/chaperone into consultation			
Gauges patient's understanding			
Gives warning shot			
Uses appropriate terminology			
Uses empathy			
Succinctly gives bad news			
Allows time for patient to react			
Checks understanding			
Provides a plan			
Offers to speak to family			
Offers follow-up, extra information sources			
Summarises			
Closes appropriately			

Offer the patient extra sources of information (e.g. clinic phone number, details on support groups, information leaflets).

Offer to speak to the patient's relatives if they consent. Make sure there is a follow-up plan in place.

Ask if the patient has any further questions (Table 3.3).

3.4 DISCHARGE LETTER

In the examination you will often be asked to write a discharge letter to the patient's general practitioner. The majority of the marks are for including straightforward details such as the patient's name, date and type of operation. It is therefore very important not to miss these easy marks. If you have written a few discharges in your career, this should not prove too difficult a task.

In the examination you will only be provided with simple details such as the patient's name and the procedure type. Otherwise the answer paper will be blank (i.e. no *pro forma*).

Here is an example of a discharge for a patient who has undergone a nasal polypectomy.

EXAMPLE 3.1 NASAL POLYPECTOMY

Bob Nash (DOB 6/1/77, Hospital No. 4234X) was admitted for endoscopic nasal polypectomy under Mr Chandra on to Ward 10 as a day case on 5 May 2016. He was discharged as planned, without complication. His pre-op CT report stated: 'Patient has had ongoing nasal obstruction for 2 years. There is bilateral nasal polyposis. All other sinuses ventilated with minimal mucosal thickening'. Mr Chandra will see Bob Nash in 4–6 weeks in clinic.

Answer

Patient:	Bob Nash
DOB:	6/1/77
Hospital No.:	4234X
Consultant:	Mr Chandra
Ward:	10
Date of admission:	5/5/16
Date of discharge:	5/5/16
Presenting complaints:	Ongoing nasal obstruction for 2 years
Diagnosis:	Nasal polyposis
Investigations:	CT sinuses – bilateral nasal polyposis
	All other sinuses ventilated with minimal mucosal thickening
Operation:	Endoscopic nasal polypectomy
Surgeon:	Mr Chandra
Complication:	No intra-operative or post-operative complications
Medications:	Given 4 weeks' saline nasal douche
	To continue with Flixonase Nasules 200 mcg bd
	With instructions on administration
	No other changes to medication
Advice:	All nasal packing removed before discharge Crusting and dry blood may cause nasal obstruction for 1–2 weeks
	Larger bleed will require readmission to hospital
	Advise 1 week off work
Follow-up:	See in clinic with histology in 4–6 weeks
Signed:	<your name> (sign and print name), CT1 to Mr Chandra (consultant ENT surgeon). GMC 7154872. Contact number: 345

3.5 OPERATION NOTE

A common question in the examination is to be asked to write an operation note for a procedure. Potentially this is a difficult station, as by its very nature it is a completely artificial situation. Rest assured the 'procedure' is usually of the nature of a tonsillectomy rather than a neck dissection.

You will only be provided with a blank sheet of paper and basic patient information:

- Patient demographics including date of birth, hospital number
- Date and time
- Operating room
- Surgeon
- Anaesthetist
- Type of anaesthesia
- Indication for procedure
- Antibiotics
- Findings
- Procedure/closure
- Post-operative instructions
- Follow-up

EXAMPLE 3.2 ADENOTONSILLECTOMY

You have just performed an adenotonsillectomy on this patient for obstructive sleep apnoea in Theatre 2. Write the operation note.
Patient: Sunil Sharma
DOB: 6/11/88
Hospital No.: 1234X
Admitted as an inpatient for overnight stay under Mr Unadkat on 5/5/16. No intra-operative or post-operative complications were recorded. The anaesthetist was Dr Beegun.

Answer

Patient:	Sunil Sharma
DOB:	6/11/88
Hospital No.:	1234X
Date:	5/5/16, 2 p.m.
Theatre:	2
Anaesthetist:	Dr Beegun
Surgeon:	\<your name>
Operation:	Adenotonsillectomy
Indication:	Obstructive sleep apnoea
Antibiotics:	None given
Findings:	Moderate adenoids, large grade 4 tonsils
Procedure:	Mouth gag
	Adenoids curetted
	Haemostasis with PNS pack
	Cold steel dissection of tonsils with ties to lower poles
	Diathermy at 15 W for haemostasis
	Teeth, temporomandibular joint, lips OK at end of procedure

Plan:	Airway and saturation monitoring overnight
	Watch for excessive swallowing and bleeding
	Eat and drink as able
	Regular analgesia
	Home tomorrow if no signs of bleeding
	No routine follow-up
Signed:	<your name> (sign and print name), CT2 to Mr Unadkat (consultant ENT surgeon). GMC 7154387. Contact number: 234

EXAMPLE 3.3 MYRINGOTOMY AND INSERTION OF GROMMETS

You have just performed bilateral myringotomies and insertion of grommets on this patient in Theatre 2 for glue ear. Write the operation note.
Patient: Alistair Carter
DOB: 6/12/07
Hospital No.: 1234X
Admitted as day case under Mrs McClenaghan on 6/5/16. No intra-operative or post-operative complications were recorded. The anaesthetist was Dr Haloob.

Answer

Patient:	Alistair Carter
DOB:	6/12/07
Hospital No.:	1234X
Date:	6/5/16, 9 a.m.
Theatre:	2
Anaesthetist:	Dr Haloob
Surgeon:	<your name>
Operation:	Bilateral myringotomies and grommet insertion
Indication:	Bilateral glue ear
Findings:	Right – flat, dull tympanic membrane with small quantity middle ear fluid
	Left – dull tympanic membrane with large middle ear effusion
Procedure:	Ear canal suctioned of wax atraumatically
	Anterior inferior myringotomies performed
	Effusions aspirated and Shah grommets inserted
	Attics clear on right and left sides
Plan:	Routine post-operative observations
	Eat and drink as able
	Home today
	Follow-up in 2 months with audiology
	Information sheet given to patient
Signed:	<your name> (sign and print name), CT2 to Mrs McClenaghan (consultant ENT surgeon). GMC 7154387. Contact number: 234

EXAMPLE 3.4 MICROLARYNGOSCOPY AND BIOPSY

You have just performed a microlaryngoscopy and biopsy on this patient in Theatre 2 for ongoing hoarseness. This revealed a small vocal cord polyp on R anterior 1/3 and 2/3 border. Write the operation note.

Patient: Huw Jones
DOB: 6/11/55
Hospital No.: 1234X
Admitted as day case under Mr George on 7/5/16. No intra-operative or post-operative complications were recorded. The anaesthetist was Dr Jacques.

Answer

Patient:	Huw Jones
DOB:	6/11/55
Hospital No.:	1234X
Date:	7/5/16, 11 a.m.
Theatre:	2
Anaesthetist:	Dr Jacques
Surgeon:	<your name>
Operation:	Microlaryngoscopy and biopsy
Indication:	Hoarseness
Antibiotics:	None given
Findings:	Small vocal cord polyp on R anterior 1/3 and 2/3 border
Procedure:	Mouthguard inserted to protect teeth
	Laryngoscopy performed
	Laryngoscope in suspension
	Microscope used to inspect cords
	Microdissection of vocal cord polyp
	1:1000 adrenaline patty used for haemostasis
	Teeth, temporomandibular joint, lips clear at end of procedure
	Specimen sent to histology
Plan:	Airway and saturation monitoring
	Eat and drink as able
	24 hours' voice rest
	Home tomorrow if well
	Follow-up in 2 weeks with histology
Signed:	<your name> (sign and print name), CT2 to Mr George (consultant ENT surgeon). GMC 7154387. Contact number: 234

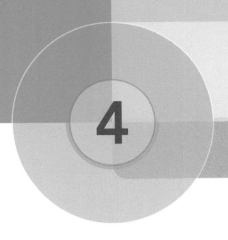

Data and Picture Interpretation Stations: Cases 1–45

4

The data and picture interpretation stations make up the majority of the stations in the examination. As we stressed in the Introduction, there are some important points to remember to ensure your success with this part of the examination. First, it is important to read the question very closely and to really make sure you specifically answer what has been asked. Second, the question often asks for a list of a certain number. For example, if it asks for three causes of a condition, you will score marks only for the first three causes that you list. Remember, if the question does not directly state how many items to list, it can often be inferred from the number of lines in the answer space. In the cases that follow we have not provided an exhaustive list of all possible answers but we have focused on the most important, as one should in the examination itself. Following the answers there is an explanatory section covering the important background and signposting the reader to areas for further reading.

DOI: 10.1201/b23029-4

CASE 1

Q1. What is the diagnosis?
Q2. List four associated symptoms.
Q3. What is the most common cause?
Q4. List four other causes.
Q5. List five investigations you may perform.
Q6. List three treatment options.

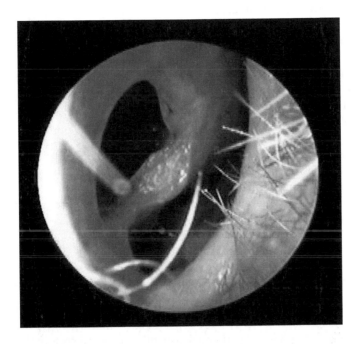

CASE 1 ANSWERS

Q1. What is the diagnosis?

Anterior nasal septal perforation

Q2. List four associated symptoms.

Nasal obstruction

Crusting

Epistaxis

Whistling

Q3. What is the most common cause?

Trauma (often nasal picking/scratching)

Q4. List four other causes.

Local trauma: Previous septal surgery, nasal cautery

Inflammatory e.g. Granulomatosis with polyangiitis (GPA), sarcoidosis

Local irritants e.g. intranasal cocaine, chemical fumes

Infections e.g. syphilis, rhinoscleroma

Neoplasia e.g. SCC, adenocarcinoma

Q5. List five investigations you may perform.

Routine blood work: FBC/U+E/ESR

c-ANCA (positive in GPA)

Angiotensin-converting enzyme (sarcoidosis)

Rheumatoid factor (elevated in rheumatoid arthritis, lupus, scleroderma)

Biopsy (to rule out malignancy)

Q6. List three treatment options.

Nasal hygiene (saline douches, 25% glucose in glycerine)

Nasal septal prosthesis (e.g. silicone button obturator)

Surgical repair (variety of local and free flap repairs, although success rates vary)

The nasal septum is a three layered structure consists of bilateral mucoperichondrium over a structural middle layer made up of the quadrangular cartilage, perpendicular plate of ethmoid or vomer. Nasal septal perforations are full thickness defects in the nasal septum. Perforations occur more commonly in the anterior septum and are more likely to be symptomatic here. Posterior perforations are often incidentally noted on rhinoscopy. Common symptoms include nasal obstruction, whistling (typical of an anterior perforation), crusting/fetor, rhinorrhoea, epistaxis and occasionally pain. They are most commonly the result of local trauma but it is important not to miss underlying systemic disease (e.g. inflammatory disease such as GPA/sarcoid), infections (syphilis, TB, fungal disease), neoplasia and intranasal drug use.

Evaluation requires careful history taking and examination and investigation as appropriate to the clinical scenario. For example, a patient presenting with a perforation after a septoplasty does not need further investigation however a new, bleeding perforation in a lifelong smoker would need biopsy to rule out malignancy.

Treatment of perforations can be divided into conservative, medical and surgical. Medical management includes providing humidification and emollients inside the nose to minimise discomfort, crusting and epistaxis. Surgical management includes the use of septal buttons and reconstructive options include the flaps such as the mucoperiochondrial and inferior turbinate flaps or auricular cartilage interposition. The larger the perforation, the lower the chance of success.

CASE 2

Q1. Describe this appearance.

Q2. What type of hearing loss would be usually associated with this condition?

Q3. List four other possible symptoms.

Q4. What would be the recommended treatment in a healthy 12-year-old?

Q5. List five complications you need to explain to the patient if this is left untreated.

Q6. List four specific complications of surgery.

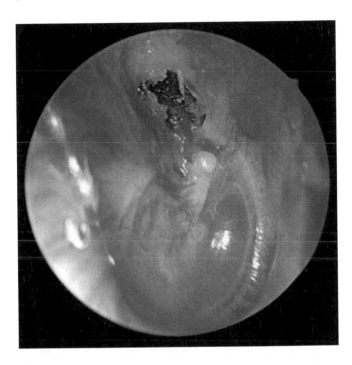

CASE 2 ANSWERS

Q1. Describe this appearance.

Attic crust (caused by cholesteatoma)

Q2. What type of hearing loss would usually be associated with this condition?

Conductive

Q3. List four other possible symptoms.

Discharge

Vertigo

Tinnitus

Facial weakness

Q4. What would be the recommended treatment in a healthy 12-year-old?

Mastoid exploration

Q5. List five complications you need to explain to the patient if this is left untreated.

Deafness

Vertigo

Facial nerve palsy

Meningitis

Intracranial abscess

Q6. List four specific complications of surgery.

Hearing loss

Vertigo

Facial nerve injury

Tinnitus

Cholesteatoma is a disease of the middle ear in which a sac of keratinising squamous epithelium grows expansively and destructively. There is a strong association with eustachian tube dysfunction although cases can also be congenital or related to chronic tympanic membrane perforation. The diagnosis is made on clinical examination (looking with magnification is important) combined with audiometry which will usually demonstrate varying degrees of conductive hearing loss depending on how much of the middle ear has been eroded. Cases can still demonstrate normal hearing though, and if the inner ear is eroded in advanced disease then a sensorineural loss can result. A CT scan is standard to provide a surgical roadmap and information around hazards and complications. The treatment is tympanomastoid surgery which may be conducted in a number of different ways (canal wall up or down, with or without obliteration, with or without ossiculoplasty) based on surgeon preference and disease extent. The risks of surgery and complications of leaving disease untreated are both related to the surrounding anatomy, so an understanding of this will help answer such questions.

CASE 3

A 34-year-old woman presents with gradual-onset bilateral hearing loss with normal tympanic membranes.

Q1. Describe the findings on this audiogram.
Q2. What is the most likely diagnosis?
Q3. List four treatment options.
Q4. What other audiometric investigation would you perform?

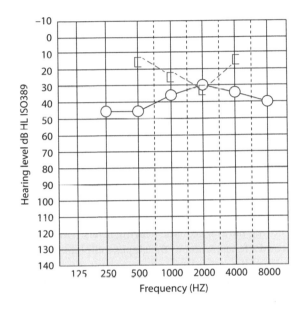

CASE 3 ANSWERS

Q1. Describe the findings on this audiogram.

Right conductive hearing loss with Carhart notch (narrowing of air-bone gap at 2000 Hz)

Q2. What is the most likely diagnosis?

Otosclerosis

Q3. List four treatment options.

Observation

Conventional hearing aid

Stapes surgery

Bone Conduction device/implant

Q4. What other audiometric investigation would you perform?

Tympanometry – Typically shows an As curve (shallow peak at approximately 0 daPa)

Otosclerosis is the commonest cause of progressive hearing loss in younger adults in the UK. There is a genetic predisposition although not all those with the disease have an affected family member or offspring. The diagnosis is made clinically: The diagnosis is made clinically, typicality an adult presenting with progressive conductive or mixed hearing loss, combined with normal otoscopy. A CT scan may help to rule out alternative causes of conductive hearing loss. Tuning fork tests also add clarity to the assessment and compliment audiometry, especially in bilateral cases where audiometric masking can prove challenging. Treatment options consist of a conventional hearing aid, stapes surgery or a bone conduction device/implant if the first two options are unacceptable. In very advanced cases, cochlear implantation may be necessary. Stapes surgery is the only option for restoring natural acoustic hearing levels. This involves fitting prosthesis between the incus and a fenestration in the stapes footplate. This carries a 0.5%–1% risk of profound sensorineural hearing loss and concurrent infection is a contraindication to surgery. Caution may also be taken in the scenario of an only-hearing ear.

CASE 4

A 60-year-old woman presents with facial weakness and a rash.

Q1. What is the likely diagnosis?
Q2. What is the aetiology?
Q3. List four associated symptoms.
Q4. List four treatment options.
Q5. List three audiometric tests for this condition.
Q6. Name a serological test for this condition.
Q7. How does the prognosis compare with an idiopathic cause (Bell palsy)?

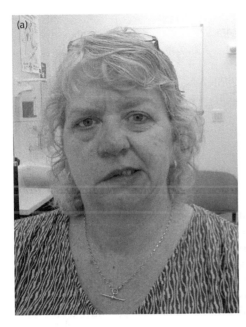

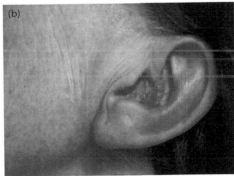

CASE 4 ANSWERS

Q1. What is the likely diagnosis?

Herpes zoster oticus (Ramsay Hunt syndrome)

Q2. What is the aetiology?

Varicella zoster infection

Q3. List four associated symptoms.

Otalgia

Hearing loss

Pharyngeal ulceration

Other cranial neuropathies

Q4. List four treatment options.

Analgesia

Eye care, e.g. eye taping and artificial tears

Corticosteroids

Aciclovir

Q5. List three audiometric tests for this condition.

Pure-tone audiogram

Acoustic reflexes

Electroneurography

Q6. Name a serological test for this condition.

Varicella zoster IgG

Q7. How does the prognosis compare with an idiopathic cause (Bell's palsy)?

The prognosis is poor in comparison with Bell's palsy

The first step in facial palsy assessment is differentiating upper motor neuron (forehead unaffected) from lower motor neuron disease (more the realm of ENT), and then grading the severity of the palsy, usually with the House-Brackmann scale (I–VI).

A common mistake is to label every facial palsy a Bell's palsy. However, this term is a diagnosis of exclusion after all other causes of lower motor neuron facial nerve palsy have been ruled out. To do this involves a history establishing time-course and associated symptoms, and an examination which includes the ears, pharynx, parotid and other lower cranial nerves. Other causes include trauma, middle ear disease, viral infections, neoplasia, neurological, autoimmune and congenital conditions. Investigations are planned accordingly, which may include audiometry, blood tests, an MRI scan and electrophysiological testing. A multidisciplinary approach is often required for persistent palsy which includes ENT, plastics, neurology, physiotherapy, speech therapy and ophthalmology.

CASE 5

Q1. What is the diagnosis?
Q2. List two possible causative organisms.
Q3. List four predisposing factors.
Q4. List four components of the management.

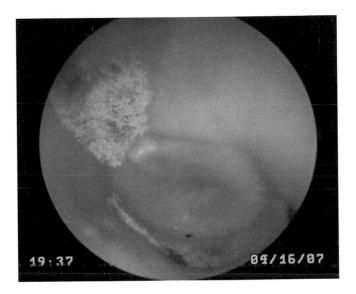

CASE 5 ANSWERS

Q1. What is the diagnosis?

Fungal otitis externa/otomycosis

Q2. List two possible causative organisms.

Aspergillus niger

Candida albicans

Actinomyces

Q3. List four predisposing factors.

Topical antibiotics

Water exposure

Canal trauma

Diabetes

Q4. List four components of the management.

Aural toilet

Topical antifungal, e.g. clotrimazole

Water precautions

Analgesia

Otitis externa is particularly common and all ENT junior doctors will have encountered many cases which require topical therapy and microsuction. Swabbing the ear for culture and sensitivities may guide choice of antibiotic drops and differentiate bacterial from fungal infection. In persistent cases, it is important not to miss an alternative diagnosis of cholesteatoma. In immunocompromised patients, with ear canal granulations and/or pain out of keeping with clinical appearance, one must also consider the possibility of necrotising otitis externa which is a potentially fatal osteomyelitis of the lateral temporal bone. Cross-sectional imaging aids diagnosis in these cases. Potential complications include venous sinus thrombosis, meningitis, intracranial abscesses and lower cranial nerve palsies. Management requires a multidisciplinary team approach and usually requires extended intravenous antibiotics via a long line.

CASE 6

The flexible nasendoscopy view of the cords is of a 45-year-old man with a weak voice. You have asked him to attempt to vocalise.

Q1. Describe the abnormality.
Q2. List two investigations you would request to determine the aetiology.
Q3. List two treatment options to improve voice quality if this is found to be idiopathic.

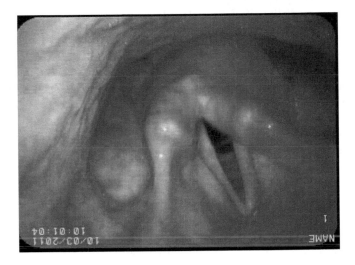

CASE 6 ANSWERS

Q1. Describe the abnormality.

Failure of medialisation of left vocal cord/left vocal cord palsy

Q2. List two investigations you would request to determine the aetiology.

Chest X-ray (CXR)

Computed tomography (CT) of the skull base to mediastinum

Q3. List two treatment options to improve voice quality if this is found to be idiopathic.

Speech and language therapy

Surgery to medialise affected vocal cord

Unilateral vocal cord paralysis presents with dysphonia (often breathy voice), dysphagia and shortness of breath. It can result from direct trauma to vocal cord (such as intubation) or secondary to damage to the recurrent laryngeal nerve e.g. by cancer, trauma or surgery. The recurrent laryngeal nerve arises from vagus nerve and courses from the brainstem through the neck and chest. Diagnosis is usually made with clinic based flexible nasendoscopy. A CT scan from the skull base to diaphragm covers the entire length of the recurrent laryngeal nerve and is an important investigation in establishing a diagnosis. Speech and language therapy can improve voice projection and pitch control. Voice quality can also be improved by surgical medialisation procedures including vocal cord injections, thyroplasty and in some instances laryngeal reinnervation procedures.

CASE 7

A 2-month-old boy presents to A&E with difficult, noisy breathing.

Q1. What is the diagnosis?
Q2. What is the classic description of the pathology shown in the picture?
Q3. List two presenting signs.
Q4. List two investigations you may perform.
Q5. List three treatment options.

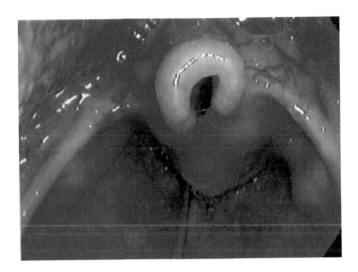

CASE 7 ANSWERS

Q1. What is the diagnosis?

Laryngomalacia

Q2. What is the classic description of the pathology shown in the picture?

Omega-shaped epiglottis

Q3. List two presenting signs.

Harsh inspiratory noises/stridor

Mild tachypnoea

Q4. List two investigations you may perform.

Laryngotracheobronchoscopy

Polysomnography

Q5. List three treatment options.

Conservative

Oxygen administration

Surgery – Supraglottoplasty, rarely tracheostomy

Laryngomalacia is the most common cause of stridor in infants. It presents within the first few weeks of life and the symptoms peak at around 6 months old and usually resolves by the end of the second year of life. It is caused by the collapse of the supraglottic structures on inspiration and causes high-pitched inspiratory stridor which typically worsens when supine or while crying. There is often a history of intermittent choking with feeding and recurrent chest infections. Severe cases result in difficulty feeding and increased metabolic expenditure on work of breathing (demonstrating tracheal tug, sternal recession and intermittent cyanosis) so that they lose significant weight and drop off centiles on growth charts. Laryngoscopy shows shortened aryepiglottic folds, an omega-shaped retroflexed epiglottis with normal vocal cord mobility and dynamic collapse of the supraglottic structures on inspiration. Most cases can be managed non-surgically with modifying feeding behaviours, encouraging upright positioning while feeding, pacing feeding with frequent burping, modifying the texture of feeds with thickener and starting treatment for reflux to reduce any laryngeal oedema. If there are signs of failure to thrive, a supraglottoplasty may be performed to widen the laryngeal inlet and reduce work of breathing.

CASE 8

A 24-year-old man presents with hearing loss following a road traffic accident.

Q1. What is this study?
Q2. What is the abnormality?
Q3. Describe what the pure-tone audiogram would very likely show.
Q4. Will the patient's hearing recover?
Q5. List five other symptoms the patient may experience.

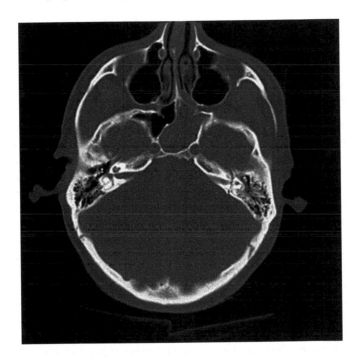

CASE 8 ANSWERS

Q1. What is this study?

Axial computed tomography (CT) of temporal bones

Q2. What is the abnormality?

Transverse fracture, left temporal bone

Q3. Describe what the pure-tone audiogram would very likely show.

Left-sided sensorineural deafness/dead ear

Q4. Will the patient's hearing recover?

No

Q5. List five other symptoms the patient may experience.

Vertigo

Facial palsy

Cerebrospinal fluid (CSF) leak

Conductive hearing loss

Tinnitus

The ENT management of temporal bone fracture usually falls secondary to ATLS resuscitation and treatment of other systemic injuries. Hearing, balance, facial nerve and CSF leak are the main considerations from our point of view. Assessment at the earliest appropriate opportunity is pertinent. On CT imaging, fractures can be divided into otic capsule involving/sparing. Alternatively, the terms longitudinal (typically a blow from the side with CSF leak more common) and transverse (higher energy from front or behind with the otic capsule more likely involved) can be used.

With regards to facial palsy, establishing the onset and severity is an important distinction. An immediate grade VI lower motor neuron palsy may require surgical exploration and repair/decompression by a skull base surgeon. Incomplete and delayed palsies should be treated with steroids.

With regards to hearing, if audiometry isn't possible then tuning fork tests may distinguish conductive from sensorineural hearing loss if the patient is conscious. Conductive losses may recover with time or be remediable with middle ear surgery at a later date. Sensorineural loss may be treated with steroids but is unlikely to recover.

CASE 9

Q1. Describe two abnormal features.
Q2. Draw and describe the associated tympanogram.
Q3. Describe the expected pure-tone audiogram.
Q4. List four management options.
Q5. List two sequelae.

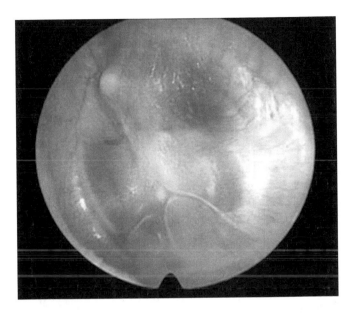

CASE 9 ANSWERS

Q1. Describe two abnormal features.
   Retracted tympanic membrane
   Fluid behind tympanic membrane

Q2. Draw and describe the associated tympanogram.
   A flat trace. This is an example tympanogram from a 4-year-old child with eustachian tube dysfunction.

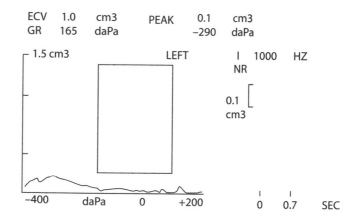

ECV 1.0 cm3   PEAK   0.1 cm3
GR   165 daPa   −290 daPa

1.5 cm3   LEFT   I 1000 HZ
                                   NR

                                   0.1 [
                                   cm3

−400   daPa   0   +200   0   0.7   SEC

Q3. Describe the expected pure-tone audiogram.
   Conductive hearing loss, particularly at low frequencies

Q4. List four management options.
   Watchful waiting
   Hearing aid
   Grommets
   Adenoidectomy

Q5. List two sequelae.
   Speech and language delay
   Acute otitis media (AOM)

Otitis Media with effusion, otherwise known as 'glue ear', is the commonest cause of new onset hearing loss in children aged 2–7, but can also affects adults. Diagnosis is made on otoscopic examination combined with flat trace (type B) tympanometry and a normal ear canal volume (0.6–2ml). Management options include hearing aids, bone conduction devices and grommet insertion, with or without adenoidectomy. It is estimated that with conservative management, 50% will resolve spontaneously at 3 months. NICE guidelines direct when surgical intervention is justified. The aim must always be to avoid prolonged auditory deprivation and the subsequent effects on speech and language development during childhood years. Certain conditions require more specific consideration due to the predisposition to more chronic effusion and hearing loss. These include Down syndrome, Cleft palate, Ciliary dyskinesias, Cranial anomalies and a history of radiotherapy. Grommets will typically be expelled spontaneously around 6–9 months. A small proportion has a resultant tympanic membrane perforation, and in others fluid re-accumulates requiring a subsequent set of grommets.

CASE 10

Q1. What is the diagnosis?
Q2. List three treatments associated with this appearance.
Q3. List two diseases associated with this appearance.
Q4. List two management strategies.

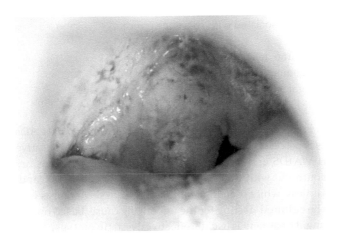

CASE 10 ANSWERS

Q1. What is the diagnosis?
Oral candidiasis

Q2. List three treatments associated with this appearance.
Systemic/inhaled corticosteroids
Systemic antibiotics
Chemotherapy/radiotherapy

Q3. List two diseases associated with this appearance.
Diabetes
Acquired immune deficiency syndrome

Q4. List two management strategies.
Oral antifungal, e.g. nystatin
Oral hygiene

Oral candidiasis is an infection of the oral cavity caused by *Candida Albicans* and in the majority of cases is associated with immunosuppression. Typical causative factors include age, diabetes, HIV/AIDS and steroid usage. Users of inhaled steroids are recommended to rinse their mouth out with water after every use. Clinically, oral candidiasis typically presents with painless, white pseudomembranous plaques. Diagnosis is generally clinical but plaques can be cultured. Testing for the underlying cause, based on the history is often required. Antifungal treatment is usually effective. Nystatin oral suspension (100000 units/mL) 5 mL orally four times daily is used first line. Fluconazole and itraconazole are indicated for severe or refractory disease.

CASE 11

Q1. In which anatomical triangle of the neck is the lesion in the photograph?
Q2. What are the four most likely diagnoses?
Q3. List three tests that could help distinguish among the possible diagnoses.
Q4. The patient is 55 years old and has no other symptoms or abnormalities on examination. The lesion appears cystic on the USS, what would you do next?
Q5. What is the embryological origin of a branchial cyst?

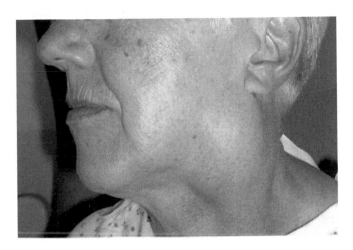

CASE 11 ANSWERS

Q1. In which anatomical triangle of the neck is the lesion in the photograph?
  Left anterior triangle

Q2. What are the four most likely diagnoses?
  Infective lymphadenopathy
  Branchial cyst
  Lymphoma
  Metastatic squamous cell carcinoma

Q3. List three tests that could help distinguish among the possible diagnoses.
  Fine needle aspiration or core biopsy (FNA; reactive, neoplastic cells, cholesterol-rich fluid in the case of branchial cysts)
  Ultrasound scan (USS; differentiate between neoplastic and reactive lymph nodes/cysts)
  Fine needle aspiration or core biopsy under USS guidance (may be reactive, neoplastic cells or cholesterol-rich fluid in the case of branchial cysts)
  Bloods, including full blood count (FBC) and C-reactive protein (e.g. to detect infective process)

Q4. The patient is 55 years old and has no other symptoms or abnormalities on examination. The FNA suggests an SCC, what would you do next?
  Arrange an MRI neck, CT thorax and a PET-CT (care coordinated by Head and Neck MDT)

Q5. What is the embryological origin of a branchial cyst?
  From the second branchial cleft

Anterior neck lumps are a common presentation. The history and examination are important in determining the cause which include infective, neoplastic, vascular e.g. carotid body tumour, inflammatory e.g. sarcoidosis, and congenital e.g. branchial cyst, lymphangioma. The first line investigation for a suspicious neck lump is USS+/- FNA. Branchial cysts are congenital masses which arise in the anterolateral neck, typically anterior to the sternocleidomastoid (SCM). When infected they can increase in size and become painful. Branchial cysts are managed by surgical resection, but it is important to recognise that cystic metastasis from a head and neck primary are a differential diagnosis. If a patient presents with metastatic neck SCC it is important to diagnose the primary site either by examination or imaging (CT/MRI/PET), as the primary site will also need treatment.

CASE 12

Q1. What is the diagnosis?
Q2. Describe three key steps in managing this patient.
Q3. Name one specific test you would perform.
Q4. What antibiotic would you not prescribe in this case?
Q5. List five indications for tonsillectomy.

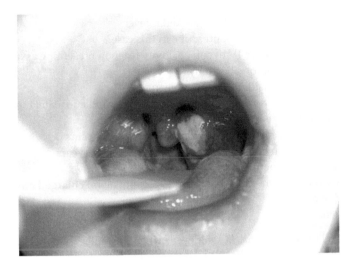

CASE 12 ANSWERS

Q1. What is the diagnosis?

Tonsillitis

Q2. Describe three key steps in managing this patient.

Analgesia and antipyretics

Antibiotics, e.g. intravenous benzylpenicillin

Intravenous fluid resuscitation

Q3. Name one specific test you would perform.

Monospot/Paul-Bunnell test for glandular fever

Q4. What antibiotic would you not prescribe in this case?

Amoxicillin (due to type IV hypersensitivity reaction presenting as a rash)

Q5. List five indications for tonsillectomy.

Recurrent severe tonsillitis for over 1 year:

Seven or more well-documented, clinically significant, adequately treated sore throats in the preceding year or

Five or more such episodes in each of the preceding 2 years or

Three or more such episodes in each of the preceding 3 years

Treatment of obstructive sleep apnoea

Diagnosis of tonsillar malignancy in cases of unilateral enlarged tonsil

Recurrent quinsy

Treatment of snoring

The pharyngeal tonsils are part of Waldeyer's ring of tonsillar tissue which also includes the adenoid tissue, tubal tonsils and lingual tonsils. Tonsillitis can be viral or bacterial. Common pathogens include adenovirus, Epstein-Barr virus, enteroviruses, and Group A beta haemolytic streptococcus (GABHS). GABHS is best treated with penicillin, and amoxicillin should be avoided as it can cause a salmon-coloured maculopapular rash if the patient has EBV. Complications of tonsillitis include peritonsillar, parapharyngeal and retropharyngeal abscesses, and systemic complications include scarlet fever, rheumatic fever and post-streptococcal glomerulonephritis.

The Paradise criteria and SIGN guidelines recommend tonsillectomy if there are seven documented episodes of tonsillitis in the preceding year, or five episodes per year for 2 consecutive years, or three documented episodes per year for 3 consecutive years. Other indications include obstructive sleep apnoea, for histological analysis or two quinsies.

Complications of tonsillectomy include pain, bleeding, infection, dental/oral injury. Primary bleeding is within 6–8 hours of surgery and secondary bleeding is typically in post-operative days 5–10).

CASE 13

Q1. What is the diagnosis?
Q2. Describe three key steps in managing this patient.
Q3. List three specific causes/precipitants for this complaint.
Q4. Name the arteries supplying the nasal septum.

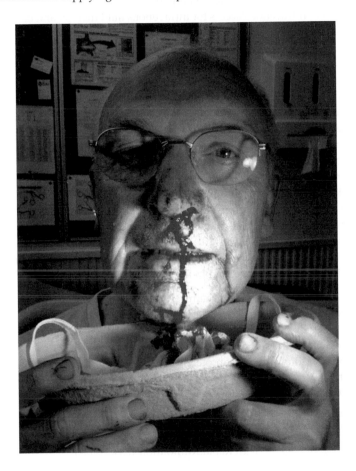

CASE 13 ANSWERS

Q1. What is the diagnosis?

Anterior epistaxis

Q2. Describe three key initial steps in managing this patient.

Patient should be managed using an Airway, Breathing, Circulation approach recognising this is a medical emergency.

1. Acquire intravenous access for intravenous fluid therapy and bloods, including FBC and group and save.
2. Control bleeding using first aid. Examine the patient and try to find a bleeding spot which could be controlled with nasal cautery, topical agents such as Floseal. Consider nasal packing (dissolvable or non-dissolvable) if required.
3. Take a full history asking specifically about risk factors (e.g. anticoagulation, trauma, bleeding diatheses).

Q3. List three specific causes/precipitants for this complaint.

Trauma

Anticoagulation

Hypertension

Q4. Name the arteries supplying the nasal septum.

Blood supply from the internal and external carotid arteries

Sphenopalatine artery and greater palatine artery (from the maxillary artery, a branch of the external carotid)

Anterior ethmoidal artery (from the ophthalmic artery from the internal carotid)

Branches of the facial artery (from the external carotid)

Epistaxis is a common topic both in clinical practice and in the exam so it is important to have a good understanding of the causes and management. Use an ABC approach recognising that patients are often elderly and can decompensate quickly.

Direct pressure on the soft part of the nose and an oral/topical ice pack are a useful first measure. You should always wear protective equipment and use a headlight and suction to examine the nose.

If the patient is bleeding despite conservative measures, consider the following in a stepwise approach:

- Cautery with $AgNO_3$ and Nasopore (or similar dissolvable packing)
- Anterior nasal packing with Rapid Rhino (non-dissolvable)
- FloSeal
- Foley Catheter + BIPP
- Surgery (e.g. SPA ligation)

CASE 14

Q1. Describe the clinical photograph.
Q2. Typically, how do patients with this type of lesion present?
Q3. List two risk factors.
Q4. Name the staging system currently in use.
Q5. List two investigations you would perform.
Q6. List three management strategies.

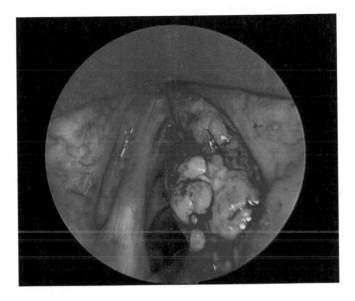

CASE 14 ANSWERS

Q1. Describe the clinical photograph.

Ulcerative growth from right vocal cord

Q2. Typically, how do patients with this type of lesion present?

Hoarse voice

Stridor in severe cases

Q3. List two risk factors.

Smoking

Excess alcohol consumption

Q4. Name the staging system currently in use.

TNM Classification for Head and Neck Cancer (Currently 8th edition)

Q5. List two investigations you would perform.

CT of the head, neck and chest

Microlaryngoscopy and biopsy

Q6. List three management strategies.

Surgery

Chemotherapy/radiotherapy

Symptom control e.g. pain relief, speech and language therapy after definitive treatment

Laryngeal cancers constitute one-third of all head and neck cancers. They often present early with voice change. Early stage disease is often curable with surgery or radiotherapy with excellent functional and oncologic outcomes. Later stage disease present with voice change pain, otalgia, swallowing difficulties, or stridor and need multimodal therapy e.g. surgery (laryngectomy) +/– chemoradiotherapy and the outcomes are poorer. All cases should be discussed at the head and neck MDT.

CASE 15

This 6-year-old girl has a recurrent lesion of the vocal cords.

Q1. Describe the clinical photograph.
Q2. Typically, how do children with this type of lesion present?
Q3. How would you manage this patient?
Q4. What is the causative agent?
Q5. Would you consider a tracheostomy in this patient?

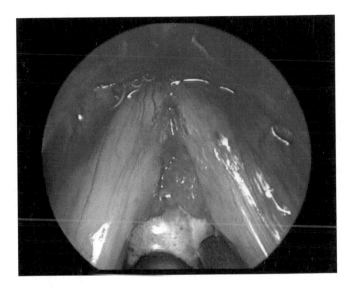

CASE 15 ANSWERS

Q1. Describe the clinical photograph.

Papilloma of the anterior commissure of the larynx

Q2. Typically, how do children with this type of lesion present?

Hoarse voice

Stridor in severe cases

Q3. How would you manage this patient?

Microlaryngoscopy

Microdebridement/laser ablation

Q4. What is the causative agent?

Human papillomavirus (types 6 and 11)

Q5. Would you consider a tracheostomy in this patient?

Tracheostomy should only be used as a last resort, as it increases the chance of disease spreading distally

Respiratory Papillomatous Virus is caused by HPV 6 and 11, with 11 causing more aggressive disease. The peak incidence is 3–5 years, and an earlier age of onset usually predicts a worse prognosis. Risk factors include maternal warts during pregnancy and laryngopharyngeal reflux. As there is a small risk of malignant transformation, the work up should include a microlaryngoscopy and biopsy to confirm the diagnosis. Management aims to improve the airway with minimal mucosal trauma for voice preservation. Surgical options include microdebrider or cold steel, as well as carbon dioxide laser however this method risks thermal damage. If patients require over 4 procedures per year, they can be offered adjuvant medical therapy in addition to surgery. This includes the Gardasil vaccine (quadrivalent vaccine given in 3 intramuscular injections) and Cidofovir (which prevents HPV DNA synthesis, and requires multiple injections into the papilloma and can achieve up to 60% cure rate).

CASE 16

Q1. What type of scan is this?
Q2. What is the most obvious abnormality?
Q3. What is the most likely diagnosis?
Q4. List three typical ways these lesions present.
Q5. List three treatment modalities.
Q6. List three alternative diagnoses.

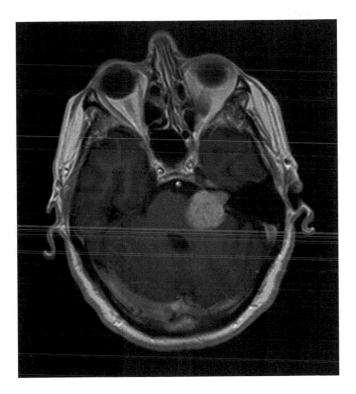

CASE 16 ANSWERS

Q1. What type of scan is this?

   Magnetic resonance imaging with gadolinium enhancement

Q2. What is the most obvious abnormality?

   Left cerebellopontine angle lesion

Q3. What is the most likely diagnosis?

   Vestibular schwannoma

Q4. List three typical ways these lesions present.

   Unilateral hearing loss

   Unilateral tinnitus

   Other cranial neuropathies, e.g. sensation changes in V nerve distribution

Q5. List three treatment modalities.

   Conservative (watch-and-wait approach)

   Surgery

   Stereotactic radiosurgery

Q6. List three alternative diagnoses.

   Meningioma

   Cholesterol granuloma

   Facial schwannoma

Asymmetric sensorineural hearing loss or tinnitus necessitates an MRI IAM scan. The vast majority return a normal result, but since benign cerebellopontine angle lesions present this way, this is the only efficient way of detecting them. Vestibular schwannoma is the commonest form of this type of lesion. Differentials include meningioma, epidermoid cyst, arachnoid cyst, facial schwannoma and cholesterol granuloma. All of these require discussion and management by the Skull Base MDT. Treatment depends on size, rate of growth and associated intracranial effects and symptoms. Some lesions will never need treatment and can be monitored via serial scanning. Of those that need intervention, options typically include surgery and cyber-knife radiotherapy, with consideration given to how much hearing there is to try and preserve when selecting mode and method.

CASE 17

Q1. What is the diagnosis?
Q2. List four ways this would typically present.
Q3. What is the aetiology of this condition?
Q4. List three treatment options.

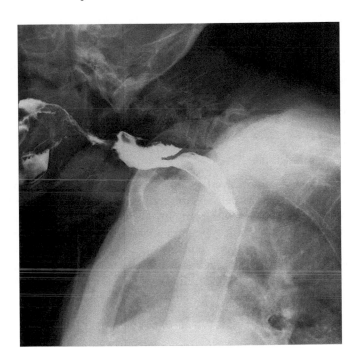

CASE 17 ANSWERS

Q1. What is the diagnosis?

Pharyngeal pouch

Q2. List four ways this would typically present.

Regurgitation

Dysphagia

Weight loss

Halitosis

Q3. What is the aetiology of this condition?

Natural weakness at Killian dehiscence between inferior constrictor and
cricopharyngeus

Q4. List three treatment options.

Conservative

Laser myotomy

Endoscopic stapling

Open surgical excision

A pharyngeal pouch is a pulsion diverticulum through the pharyngeal mucosa via Killian's dehiscence, a natural weakness between the fibres of cricopharyngeus and thryopharyngeus. Patients are often elderly with co-morbidities. It is therefore important to take a full history focussing on weight loss, regurgitation, chest infections and aspiration. It is important not to miss any red flag symptoms e.g. pain/neck lumps/otalgia. All patients should have flexible nasendoscppy performed and a contrast swallow arranged. In the UK if trans-oral access is possible the first line treatment is endoscopic stapling with other methods used in difficult or more complicated cases.

CASE 18

Q1. What is the abnormality pictured here?
Q2. Name two common tumours in this gland.
Q3. List two symptoms that would concern you about malignancy.
Q4. List two investigations you would perform.
Q5. List three things you would warn the patient about if you were considering surgical removal of the lump.

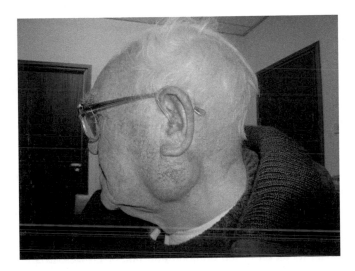

CASE 18 ANSWERS

Q1. What is the abnormality pictured here?

Left parotid lump

Q2. Name two common tumours in this gland.

Pleomorphic adenoma

Warthin's tumour

Q3. List two symptoms that would concern you about malignancy.

Facial nerve palsy

Pain

Q4. List two investigations you would perform.

Ultrasound

Ultrasound guided FNA

(Other imaging, e.g. CT/MRI may be indicated depending on presentation)

Q5. List three things you would warn the patient about if you were considering surgical removal of the lump.

Bleeding/haematoma formation

Facial nerve injury

Frey's syndrome (gustatory sweating)

Salivary gland tumours can occur in the parotid, submandibular gland, sublingual gland, and minor salivary glands. There are wide variety of possible histological subtypes both benign (e.g. pleomorphic adenoma, Warthin's) and malignant (e.g. mucoepidermoid, acinic cell, adenoid cystic). Both benign and malignant tumours can present as painless, fixed masses.

History should focus on onset, duration and rate of growth. It is important to ask about facial weakness or pain. Treatment of benign tumours is typically surgical excision whereas malignant tumours may require surgical excision +/− neck dissection +/− chemo-radiotherpy depending on grade and stage of tumour.

CASE 19

Q1. What is the most likely diagnosis?
Q2. List three risk factors.
Q3. List two investigations you would perform.
Q4. List three management strategies.

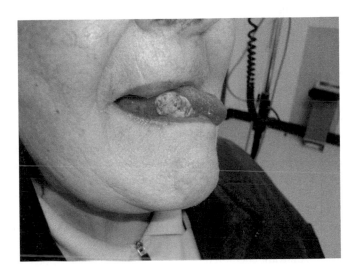

CASE 19 ANSWERS

Q1. What is the most likely diagnosis?

Right-sided tongue squamous cell carcinoma

Q2. List three risk factors

Smoking

Excessive alcohol consumption

Betel nut chewing

Q3. List two investigations you would perform.

Staging CT of the head, neck, chest (MRI useful for head and neck soft tissues)

Biopsy

Q4. List three management strategies.

Surgical excision and reconstruction e.g. forearm free flap, neck dissection

Chemotherapy/radiotherapy

Palliation

Oral cancer arises from the mucosa of the oral cavity. Squamous cell carcinomas account for over 90% of these cancers. Early cancers present as white or red patches of the mucosa which can then ulcerate and bleed. Patients should be carefully examined for concurrent tumours and spread to the neck. Biopsy and imaging with CT/MRI form the mainstay of investigations. Tumour, Node, Metastasis (TNM) staging is used plan treatment and inform prognosis. Surgical excision is the primary treatment which may involve reconstruction of the defect. Neck dissection is often required because of the high chance of metastatic spread. Adjuvant chemoradiotherapy can have complications both short term, such as mucositis, and longer term such as osteoradionecrosis. All patients should be managed with an MDT approach.

CASE 20

Q1. Name the structures labelled A–F.
Q2. What is the major cation in A?
Q3. Which compartment (A–F) does the oval window open to?
Q4. Name the point where the scala vestibuli and scala tympani meet.
Q5. What is the modiolus?
Q6. Which compartment is involved in Ménière syndrome?

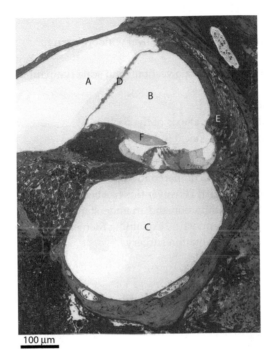

100 μm

CASE 20 ANSWERS

Q1. Name the structures labelled A–F.
    A: Scala vestibuli
    B: Scala media
    C: Scala tympani
    D: Reissner's membrane
    E: Stria vascularis
    F: Tectorial membrane

Q2. What is the major cation in A?
    Sodium

Q3. Which compartment (A–F) does the oval window open to?
    A

Q4. Name the point where the scala vestibuli and scala tympani meet.
    Helicotrema

Q5. What is the modiolus?
    The conical-shaped central axis of the cochlea

Q6. Which compartment is involved in Meniere's disease?
    B

This is a slightly unusual topic compared to other stations. After all you're training to be a surgeon, not a histopathologist! However this has been known to come up many times in the MRCS (ENT) OSCE examination and an understanding of cochlear anatomy becomes important in hearing loss diagnostics, explaining Meniere's disease to patients, and in the finer aspects of cochlear implantation surgery.

CASE 21

Q1. What is this imaging modality?
Q2. What is the obvious abnormality?
Q3. List three treatment options.
Q4. List three specific complications of surgery to the gland.

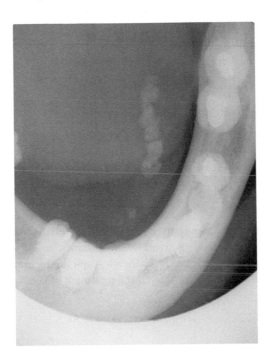

CASE 21 ANSWERS

Q1. What is this imaging modality?
   Plain X-ray of the floor of mouth
Q2. What is the obvious abnormality?
   Left submandibular salivary duct stone
Q3. List three treatment options
   Symptomatic, e.g. increased fluid intake and analgesia
   Sialoendoscopy and basket retrieval of stone
   Surgical removal of gland
Q4. List three specific complications of surgery to the gland.
   Weakness of lip (damage to marginal mandibular nerve)
   Hematoma/seroma
   Weakness of tongue

Sialolithiasis is defined as the formation of stones in the major salivary glands (submandibular, parotid, sublingual glands). It is a common cause of salivary gland swelling. Obstructed salivary glands can become inflamed and infected and occasionally abscesses can form, the first line investigation for patients presenting with suspected salivary gland stone is an ultrasound of the gland and neck which can also exclude salivary gland tumours. Plain films were the initial choice in the past and are still used in some settings. If available, sialography may also be used as this can be both diagnostic and therapeutic (in the case of small stones). If medical treatment (massage/silaogogues/NSAIDs and antibiotics as required) is not successful, then sialoendoscopy can be used for stones up to 4mm. Surgical excision of the gland is considered the treatment of last resort but is definitive.

CASE 22

This is a photograph from an endoscopic intranasal operation.

Q1. What is the diagnosis?
Q2. List two presenting symptoms.
Q3. List two medical treatments.
Q4. If this patient also reported 'a wheezy chest', what medication would you advise them
to avoid?
Q5. List three main complications of surgical removal.

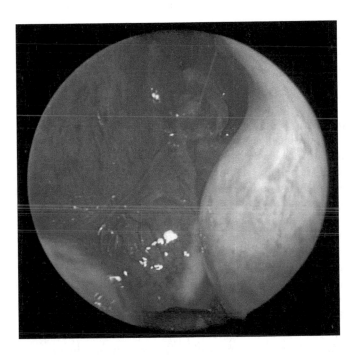

CASE 22 ANSWERS

Q1. What is the diagnosis?

Nasal polyp

Q2. List two presenting symptoms.

Nasal obstruction

Anosmia

Q3. List two medical treatments.

Intranasal steroids

Systemic steroids

Q4. If this patient also reported 'a wheezy chest', what medication would you advise them to avoid?

Aspirin (this may represent Samter's triad)

Q5. List three main complications of surgical removal.

Bleeding

Risk to vision

CSF leak

Nasal polyps are a common presentation to ENT outpatients. They have a 4:1 M:F predominance with an incidence of 1–20:1000, and are associated with late onset asthma. Symptoms include a blocked nose, runny nose, poor sense of smell or taste, and catarrh.

Nasal polyps are benign swellings inside the nose which often originate from the ethmoid sinuses. They contain inflammatory fluid but over two-thirds do not have systemic allergic symptoms.

Samter's triad of nasal polyps, asthma, and aspirin hypersensitivity is seen in 8% of polyp patients, and they are more at risk of polyp recurrence.

Unilateral polyps are rare and therefore always need further investigations. Polyps are also rare in children and therefore cystic fibrosis should be considered.

Polyps may shrink with nasal steroids, and newer nasal steroids can safely be used for many years with low systemic absorption. Oral steroids have good effect but more significant systemic side effects. However, in medication resistant disease, surgical polypectomy is required. They will often still require topical treatment post-operatively to reduce recurrence. Combining the polypectomy with endoscopic sinus surgery can elongate time to recurrence but approximately 75% will get recurrence with average time to recurrence of 4 years.

5–10% patients undergoing FESS will experience minor complications such as mild haemorrhage or infection, with only 0.5% experiencing major complications including orbital injury, CSF leak and severe haemorrhage.

CASE 23

Thyroid-stimulating hormone, 23 (0.4–3.0) Free T4, 1.1 (0.8–1.8)
Total T3, 159 (80–180) Thyroglobulin, 28 (<35)
Thyroid peroxidase antibodies, 675 (<45)

Q1. What is the diagnosis?
Q2. List two tests to help confirm the diagnosis.
Q3. List five typical presenting symptoms of hypothyroidism.
Q4. Name the most common medical treatment.
Q5. What are two indications for surgery?

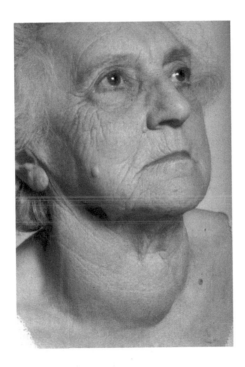

CASE 23 ANSWERS

Q1. What is the diagnosis?
   Hashimoto thyroiditis
Q2. List two tests to help confirm the diagnosis.
   USS
   Detection of elevated levels of antithyroid peroxidase antibodies
Q3. List five typical presenting symptoms of hypothyroidism.
   Weight gain
   Voice change
   Loss of hair
   Cold intolerance
   Muscle weakness
Q4. Name the most common medical treatment.
   Thyroid hormone replacement
Q5. What are two indications for surgery?
   Any risk of malignancy
   Mass effect causing airway compromise

Hypothyroidism results from low levels of thyroid hormone. The most common cause of hypothyroidism in the UK is Hashimoto's thyroiditis. Iodine deficiency remains an important cause in some geographic regions. Other causes include drugs e.g. amiodarone, radiotherapy, thyroid surgery and pituitary disease.

Signs and symptoms can be mild and non-specific. Typical features include cold intolerance, decreased sweating, skin changes and fatigue.

Serum TSH level is used to screen for primary hypothyroidism. In overt hypothyroidism, TSH levels are raised with low levels of free T4. Levels of anti-thyroid antibodies such as the thyroid peroxidase antibodies should also be evaluated.

Hypothyroidism is mainly treated with levothyroxine monotherapy. Severe hypothyroidism is an endocrine emergency requiring specialist medical care.

The most common causes of hyperthyroidism are Graves' disease and toxic multinodular goitre. Hyperthyroidism may present with weight loss, palpitations, anxiety, weakness, diarrhoea and fatigue. Evaluation for TSH, free T4 and anti TSH antibody should be performed. Treatment will be coordinated by endocrinology and includes medical (beta blockers, thioamide drugs e.g. carbimazole, and radioactive iodine) or surgical e.g. total thyroidectomy.

CASE 24

Q1. What is the abnormality pictured here?
Q2. List two presenting symptoms.
Q3. What is the staging system used?
Q4. What is the tissue of origin of this lesion?
Q5. List three management strategies.

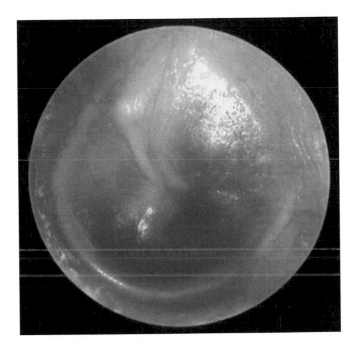

CASE 24 ANSWERS

Q1. What is the abnormality pictured here?

Glomus tympanicum (paraganglioma)

Q2. List two presenting symptoms.

Conductive hearing loss

Pulsatile tinnitus

Q3. What is the staging system used?

Fisch classification

Q4. What is the tissue of origin of this lesion?

Neuroendocrine tissue

Q5. List three management strategies.

Observation with repeat scanning

Stereotactic radiosurgery

Surgical resection

Paragangliomas are tumours of the middle ear and skull base that arise from chemoreceptor tissue associated with the autonomic nervous system. They are supplied by the ascending pharyngeal artery and there are 4 types: Glomus tympanicum, Glomus vagale, Glomus jugulare and Carotid Body tumours (the commonest). Patients may present with conductive hearing loss, pulsatile tinnitus or a mass in the ear or neck. The most destructive cases can cause lower cranial nerve palsies and Horner's syndrome. Genetics play a role and screening exists for high-risk groups with a number of genes identified. Management at the skull base multidisciplinary team is mandated for all cases. MRI, CT & PET scans are all part of the diagnostic workup. Malignant potential is rare but possible. Treatment options include serial monitoring, radiotherapy, subtotal resection and radical tympanomastoid/neck surgery.

CASE 25

Q1. What is the structure labelled A? Name a ligament and a muscle that attach here.
Q2. What is the structure labelled B? List two muscles that attach here.
Q3. What is the structure labelled C? List four structures that pass through this structure.
Q4. What is the structure labelled D? Name a structure that passes through this structure.

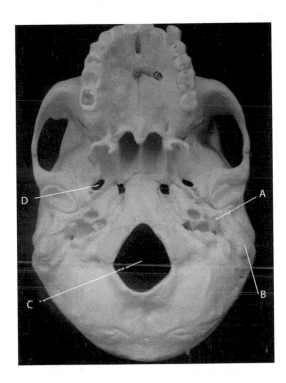

CASE 25 ANSWERS

Q1. What is the structure labelled A? Name a ligament and a muscle that attach here.
  Styloid process
  Styloglossus muscle
  Stylohyoid ligament

Q2. What is the structure labelled B? List two muscles that attach here.
  Mastoid process
  Sternocleidomastoid
  Posterior belly of digastric

Q3. What is the structure labelled C? List four structures that pass through this structure.
  Foramen magnum
  Spinal cord
  Meninges
  Vertebral arteries
  Spinal root of cranial nerve XI

Q4. What is the structure labelled D? Name a structure that passes through this structure.
  Foramen ovale
  Mandibular division of cranial nerve V

Foramina	Nerve	Vessels	Other
Cribriform foramina in cribriform plate	I Olfactory nerve (with bulb lying above) Anterior ethmoidal nerves		
Optic canal	II Optic nerve	Ophthalmic artery	
Superior orbital fissure	III Oculomotor nerve (superior and inferior divisions) V_1 (ophthalmic division of the trigeminal nerve; divided into lacrimal, frontal, nasocilliary branches) IV Abducent nerve VI Trochlear nerve	Superior ophthalmic vein Branch of inferior ophthalmic vein	
Foramen rotundum	V_2 (maxillary division of the trigeminal nerve)	Artery of foramen rotundum, emissary veins	
Foramen ovale	V_3 (mandibular division of the trigeminal nerve), lesser petrosal nerve	Accessory meningeal artery, emissary veins	Otic ganglion lies just below

Foramen spinosum	Meningeal branch of V$_3$	Middle meningeal artery and vein	
Foramen lacerum		NB ICA exits, but does not pass through it	
Internal auditory meatus	VII Facial nerve VIII Vestibulocochlear nerve	Labyrinthine artery	Vestibular ganglion
Jugular foramen	IX Glossopharyngeal nerve X Vagal nerve XI Accessory nerve	Inferior petrosal sinus joins sigmoid sinus and forms jugular bulb before becoming external jugular vein Meningeal branches of occipital and ascending pharyngeal arteries	
Hypoglossal canal	XII Hypoglossal canal		
Foramen magnum	Spinal cord (medulla) XI Spinal part of the Accessory nerve (ascends to join cranial part to exit jugular foramen)	Vertebral arteries Anterior and posterior spinal arteries Dural veins	Meninges

CASE 26

Q1. What is this investigation?
Q2. What are the abnormalities shown?
Q3. List three typical symptoms this patient may present with.
Q4. List five risks of endoscopic surgery for this condition.
Q5. If damaged, which vessel can cause a rise in intraorbital pressure?

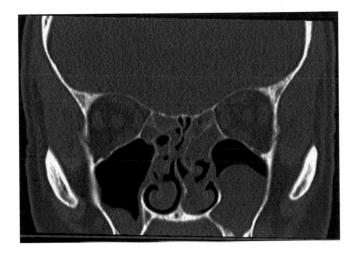

CASE 26 ANSWERS

Q1. What is this investigation?

    CT paranasal sinuses

Q2. What are the abnormalities shown?

    Opacification of the left maxillary and ethmoid sinuses

Q3. List three typical symptoms this patient may present with.

    Rhinorrhoea

    Nasal obstruction

    Anosmia

Q4. List five risks of endoscopic surgery for this condition.

    Bleeding

    Infection

    Damage to vision

    CSF leak

    Meningitis

Q5. If damaged, which vessel can cause a rise in intraorbital pressure?

    Anterior ethmoidal artery

EPOS 2020 publishes very useful information about the diagnosis and management of chronic rhinosinusitis (CRS), https://epos2020.com/Documents/supplement_29.pdf.

They define CRS if there are two or more of the following symptoms, one of which should be **nasal obstruction** and/or **discoloured discharge**

    +/– facial pain/pressure

    +/– reduction or loss of smell

    For >12 weeks

Alarm symptoms that require early escalation and further investigation include signs of sepsis or meningitis, eye signs, visual changes, severe headaches, neurological symptoms, bleeding, crusting, unilateral symptoms or cacosmia.

Patients should initially be managed with self-education and self-care, including saline rinses and over the counter intra-nasal corticosteroids (INCS) for 6–12 weeks. If there is no demonstrated improvement primary care should offer education about technique and compliance with saline rinses and INCS; and consider oral corticosteroids (OCS). If there is still no improvement, secondary care can arrange additional work up, including nasendoscopy to look for polyps and mucopurulent discharge, a skin prick test, laboratory testing including IgE and white blood cell differential (looking for eosinophilia), and a CT scan. If the CT scan shows blocked osteomeatal complexes (OMC) +/– polyps, then a functional endoscopic sinus surgery may help improve their symptoms.

CASE 27

Q1. What is the obvious pathology?
Q2. What is your advice to the referring A&E officer?
Q3. What is the management if this patient is not seen until 3 months after the injury?

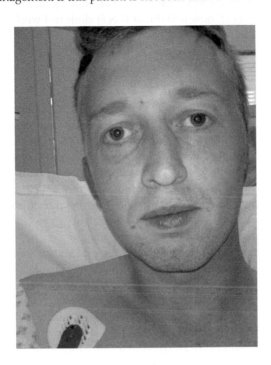

CASE 27 ANSWERS

Q1. What the obvious pathology?

Fractured nasal bones

Q2. What is your advice to the referring A&E officer?

If no other injuries, no septal haematoma and no ongoing epistaxis, the patient can be seen in the ear, nose and throat (ENT) clinic in 1 week when the swelling has subsided.

Q3. What is the management if this patient is not seen until 3 months after the injury?

It is most likely that the bones will have healed and, therefore, will need a septorhinoplasty under general anaesthesia.

The nasal bones comprise the upper third of the external nose. In head or facial trauma there may be other injuries that take priority (e.g. intracranial bleed/complex facial fractures).

Traumatic epistaxis can be brisk and can be difficult to control. The anterior ethmoid artery is more commonly involved in traumatic epistaxis, and may require more significant intervention e.g. posterior pack with Foley catheter and anterior BIPP packing +/– anterior ethmoid ligation (typically undertaken external via a Lynch incision).

Nasal trauma patients need to be examined for a septal haematoma: commonly in the anterior septum and appear as red, usually bilateral, boggy swellings in the nasal cavity. These require urgent attention as they risk stripping the perichondrium off cartilage and consequential cartilage necrosis which leads to a septal perforation and change of shape of the nose. If septal haematomas are not drained in a timely manner, they could develop into a septal abscess which carries a higher likelihood of necrosis and perforation, but also risks infection tracking intracranially due to the rich valveless venous complex of the septum and causing intracranial complications including septic cavernous thrombosis.

Ideally nasal fracture patients are reviewed at 7–10 days once the swelling has reduced to facilitate formal assessment of any nasal bone deviation by palpation, and a manipulation under anaesthetic (MUA) can be offered if necessary. MUA are frequently performed under local anaesthetic, unless the patient is young or suffers with behavioural issues, or if there are depressed segments that require elevation. They are frequently performed in clinic with topical agents (e.g. lidocaine) on cotton pledgets inside the nose, and lignospan injected along the lateral aspects of the nasal bones and premaxilla, targeting the infra-orbital, infratrochlear and dorsal nasal nerves. Depressed segments need elevating with a Hill's elevator or Walsham forceps. It is useful to note that a MUA cannot correct septal deviations: These will require a formal septo(+/– rhino-)plasty once everything has healed (at least 6–8 months post-injury).

CASE 28

Q1. What is the obvious pathology?
Q2. List four ways the patient may have presented.
Q3. What is the staging system currently in use?
Q4. List three treatment modalities.

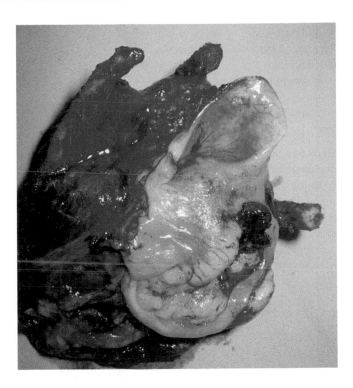

CASE 28 ANSWERS

Q1. What is the obvious pathology?

Right pyriform fossa ulcerative lesion

Q2. List four ways the patient may have presented.

Weight loss

Dysphagia

Odynophagia

Referred otalgia

Q3. What is the staging system currently in use?

TMN (8th edition)

Q4. List three treatment modalities.

Surgery

Chemotherapy/radiotherapy

Palliation

The hypopharynx between the lower end of the oropharynx and the oesophageal inlet is divided into the post cricoid, piriform fossa and posterior pharyngeal wall subsites with the piriform fossa the most commonly affected. The vast majority of cancers arising in this region are squamouis cell carcinomas. Tumours often present late commonly with pain, neck lumps and dysphagia and bleeding. The key investigations are pharyngoscopy and biopsy and MRI/CT neck and CT chest for staging. Management is either primary chemo-radiotherapy or surgical in the form of total pharyngectomy and laryngectomy with neck dissection with adjuvant chemoradiotherapy.

CASE 29

Q1. Which audiogram best fits with glue ear?
Q2. Which audiogram best fits with otosclerosis?
Q3. Which audiogram best fits with presbycusis?
Q4. Which audiogram would benefit most from cochlear implantation?
Q5. Which audiogram best fits with noise-induced hearing loss?
Q6. Which audiogram best fits with Ménière syndrome?

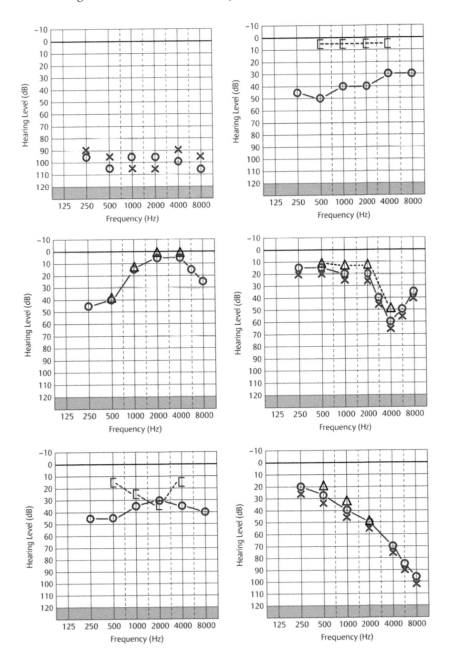

CASE 29 ANSWERS

Q1. Which audiogram best fits with glue ear?

   B

Q2. Which audiogram best fits with otosclerosis?

   E

Q3. Which audiogram best fits with presbycusis?

   F

Q4. Which audiogram would benefit most from cochlear implantation?

   A

Q5. Which audiogram best fits with noise-induced hearing loss?

   D

Q6. Which audiogram best fits with Ménière syndrome?

   C

Being comfortable with audiometric interpretation is a crucial entry-level skill in ENT. Make yourself familiar with the symbols for unmasked bone conduction, as well as air conduction and masked bone conduction for the left and right ears.

Once you've done that, then be able to tell a conductive (air-bone gap) from a sensori-neural (no air-bone gap) hearing loss (when thresholds are lower than 20dB).

Then make yourself familiar with different 'classic patterns'. Note that these patterns are not diagnostic. Otosclerosis does not always feature a Carhart notch. Noise-induced hearing loss does not always feature a notch. But knowing these patterns help counsel patients appropriately in the context of their history and examination.

At a more advanced level, masking is the next topic to understand. Because sounds played into one side of the head may be heard in the other ear, there are specific circumstances where a distracting sound, known as masking, must be used in the non-test ear to gain an accurate test. Ask your local audiology colleague to explain to you the 'rules of masking'. That will also help you to understand why there is such a thing as a 'maximal conductive hearing loss' and how to spot potential 'non-organic' hearing losses.

CASE 30

Q1. List four objects used in the management of epistaxis.
Q2. Name object D.
Q3. Name object F.
Q4. What does the acronym BIPP stand for?

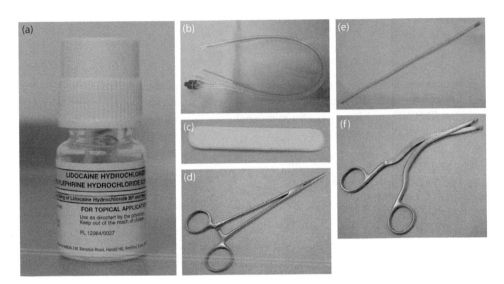

CASE 30 ANSWERS

Q1. List four objects used in the management of epistaxis.

A (Lidocaine + Phenylephrine spray), B (Foley catheter), C (Merocel nasal pack) and E (Silver nitrate cautery)

Q2. Name object D.

Birkett straight forceps

Q3. Name object F.

Tonsil grasping forceps

Q4. What does the acronym BIPP stand for?

Bismuth iodoform paraffin paste

Each unit will have their own guidelines, but the ENT UK guidelines published in 2019 can be found here: https://www.entuk.org/rhinology-and-facial-plastics-guidelines (accessible via the ENT UK guidelines page for members).

The basic ladder is as follows:

First Aid
- Anterior nasal pressure
- Head forwards
- Ice pack

Anterior rhinoscopy
- Clean with co-phenylcaine soaked cotton wool
- If visible vessel, apply silver nitrate cautery / electrocautery

Medical adjuncts
- Analgesia +/- stat antihypertensive
- If anticoagulated, consider reversal
- If difficult to control bleed, consider Tranexamic Acid

Anterior packing
- If low-flow, insert soft dissolvable pack (eg nasopore) or consider Floseal
- If high-flow, insert rigid non-dissolvable pack (to be removed after 24-48hr)

Posterior packing
- If still bleeding, consider posterior pack

Surgical intervention
- If still bleeding consider Sphenopalatine Artery Ligation
- If traumatic bleed, consider Anterior Ethmoid Artery Ligation
- If uncontrollable, consider External Carotid Artery ligation *(rare)*

Adjuncts
- Interventional Radiology may be able to perform coiling or embolisation

CASE 31

Q1. List four objects used in tonsillectomy.
Q2. Name object B.
Q3. Name object D.
Q4. Name object F.

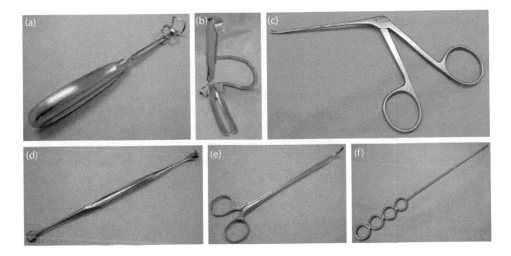

CASE 31 ANSWERS

Q1. List four objects used in tonsillectomy.

B (Boyle-Davis gag), D (Mollison pillar retractor), E (curved Negus) and F (Draffin rod)

Q2. Name object B.

Boyle-Davis gag

Q3. Name object D.

Mollison pillar retractor

Q4. Name object F.

Draffin rod

The instruments pictured are used for the set up and positioning for tonsillectomies regardless of the technique. There are several accepted techniques and surgeons often have their own personal preference. Choice of technique should be ideally based on personal complication rates and disclosed to the patients during the consenting process, or departmental/ national complication rates if that data is unavailable. Different techniques were evaluated and discussed in the National Prospective Tonsillectomy Audit (NPTA) published in 2005, https:// www.rcseng.ac.uk/library-and-publications/rcs-publications/docs/tonsillectomy-audit/.

These were the bleed rates quoted in the NPTA.

Surgical technique	Post-operative haemorrhage rate (%)	Total return to theatre rate (%)
Cold steel tonsillectomy	1.3	1.0
Cold dissection with diathermy haemostasis	2.9	1.7
Bipolar diathermy	3.9	2.4
Monopolar diathermy	6.1	4.0
Coblation	4.4	3.1

Their recommendations included

- 'Hot' techniques should be used with caution especially when used as a dissection tool.
- Surgeons using monopolar diathermy should consider using an alternative technique as there are no advantages to using it over other methods.

NB they did not differentiate between intra- and extra-capsular coblation.

In 2019 Getting It Right First Time (GIRFT) published data which found much higher readmission rates than the NPTA, especially in adults. They looked specifically at intra-capsular coblation tonsillectomy and found a very low complication rate, with 0.4% post-operative haemorrhage rate, with none requiring surgical arrest. They found 2.4% required secondary revision surgery to remove remnant tonsil tissue, https://gettingitrightfirsttime. co.uk/wp-content/uploads/2019/12/ENT-Report-Nov19-M.pdf.

Patient group	NPTA Post-operative haemorrhage rate (%)	NPTA Total return to theatre rate (%)	GIRFT Post-operative haemorrhage rate (%)	GIRFT Total return to theatre rate (%)
Combined adult and children	3.5	0.8	8.0	1.3
Adult	4.9	1.2	13.0	2.3

CASE 32

Q1. Which instrument is most appropriately used to remove an inhaled foreign body?
Q2. Which instrument is most appropriately used to remove an oesophageal foreign body?
Q3. Which instruments are most appropriately used to remove a foreign body from an ear?
Q4. Name object G.

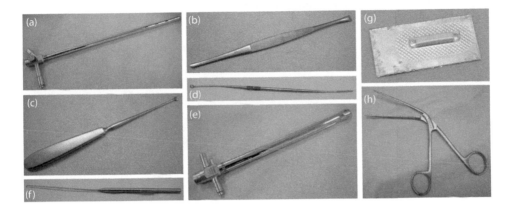

CASE 32 ANSWERS

Q1. Which instrument is most appropriately used to remove an inhaled foreign body?
A (ventilating bronchoscope)

Q2. Which instrument is most appropriately used to remove an oesophageal foreign body?
E (rigid oesophagoscope)

Q3. Which instruments are most appropriately used to remove a foreign body from an ear?
D (Jobson-Horne probe) and F (wax hook)

Q4. Name object G.
Pope wick

CASE 33

Q1. What is this?
Q2. What is its most common use in ENT?
Q3. List two consequences of this being inserted into the nasal cavity.
Q4. List two consequences of this being inserted into the ear of a child.
Q5. List three investigations you would perform for an adult with learning disabilities reported to have ingested this 2 hours ago.
Q6. If presence were confirmed at the level of the cricopharyngeus, what would you do?
Q7. What is the most serious risk of this procedure?

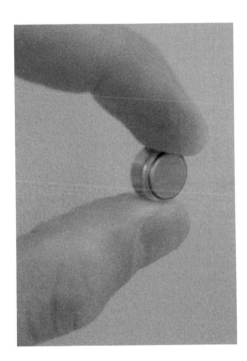

CASE 33 ANSWERS

Q1. What is this?

Watch battery

Q2. What is its most common use in ENT?

Hearing aid

Q3. List two consequences of this being inserted into the nasal cavity.

Chemical burn to nasal mucosa

Septal perforation

Q4. List two consequences of this being inserted into the ear of a child.

Chemical burn to external auditory canal

Deafness

Q5. List three investigations you would perform for an adult with learning disabilities reported to have ingested this 2 hours ago.

Erect CXR

Lateral soft tissue neck X-ray

Abdominal X-ray

Q6. If presence were confirmed at the level of the cricopharyngeus, what would you do?

Urgent rigid oesophagoscopy for removal

Q7. What is the most serious risk of this procedure?

Perforated oesophagus

Button batteries are single-cell batteries in which the positive and negative terminals are insulated from one another. They are often used in watches and car keys and resemble buttons or coins. If accessible to children, they will frequently place them in their ears, nose or mouth and swallow or inhale them. When the battery is surrounded by bodily fluids, a circuit is created which can release a strong alkali which causes corrosive burns, and therefore they need to be urgently removed. Within two hours a swallowed battery can cause an oesophageal perforation.

CASE 34

Q1. What is the abnormality pictured here?
Q2. List two associated symptoms.
Q3. What is the most common aetiology?
Q4. List two management strategies.
Q5. Name one measure the patient could take to prevent progression.

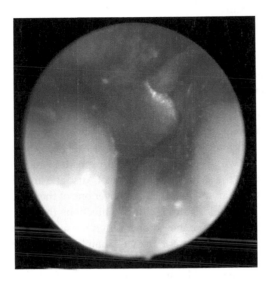

CASE 34 ANSWERS

Q1. What is the abnormality pictured here?

Bony exostoses of the auditory canal

Q2. List two associated symptoms.

Deafness

Wax impaction

Q3. What is the most common aetiology?

Cold-water exposure

Q4. List two management strategies.

No treatment if asymptomatic

Surgical bony meatoplasty

Q5. Name one measure the patient could take to prevent progression.

Use earplugs when swimming

Concentric narrowing of the external auditory canal maybe bony or due to soft tissue fibrosis. In terms of bony narrowing, the main differentials are exostoses and osteomas.

Exostoses are usually multiple, bilateral and consist of broad based bony protuberances. There is an association with repeated cold water exposure which is why this condition is more commonly seen in the surfing populations of Australia and USA.

Osteomas to be singular and pedunculated over one of the bony suture lines.

Both may cause hearing loss and recurrent infections through the trapping of debris and obstruction of the tympanic membrane. Often no surgical treatment is required but if symptoms become very problematic then a canalplasty can be performed to surgically widen the ear canal with a drill. Care must be taken not to injure the tympanic membrane or the facial nerve. New ear canal skin may need to be grafted.

CASE 35

Q1. What is the abnormality pictured here?
Q2. List three presenting symptoms.
Q3. What is the most common aetiology?
Q4. List two management options.
Q5. List three complications that can occur as a result of this condition.

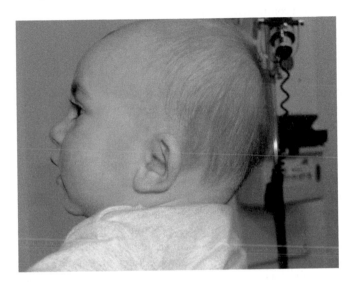

CASE 35 ANSWERS

Q1. What is the abnormality pictured here?

Left acute mastoiditis

Q2. List three presenting symptoms.

Otalgia

Fever

Ear discharge

Q3. What is the most common aetiology?

AOM

Q4. List two management options.

Intravenous antibiotics

Cortical mastoidectomy

Q5. List three complications that can occur as a result of this condition.

Sigmoid sinus thrombosis

Intracranial abscess

Meningitis

Mastoiditis is a complication of acute otitis media, for which children tend to be more susceptible. Identification of pinna protrusion, post-aural erythema, tenderness or fluctuance should prompt the consideration of admission for intravenous antibiotics. Further complications include intracranial sepsis, spread to the neck and temple, and facial nerve palsy. Surgery may be required in the case of complications, systemic toxicity or failure to improve with medical treatment. A CT scan should be performed prior to any surgery to exclude concomitant intracranial sepsis. Surgical intervention may comprise mastoidectomy with or without grommet insertion. Underlying causative factors such as immunodeficiency or the presence of cholesteatoma may sometimes be implicated.

CASE 36

Q1. Describe this picture.
Q2. What other radiological signs can be associated with this presentation?
Q3. What would your management be?
Q4. What signs and symptoms would make you concerned about a perforation?
Q5. What would your management of a perforation be?

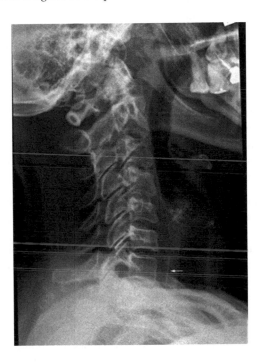

CASE 36 ANSWERS

Q1. Describe this picture.

Lateral soft tissue neck radiograph (X-ray) showing a foreign body at the level of C7

Q2. What other radiological signs can be associated with this presentation?

Loss of cervical lordosis

Air fluid level

Widened pre-vertebral shadow

Subcutaneous emphysema

Q3. What would your management be?

Nil by mouth, discuss with anaesthetist on call, emergency theatre coordinator and ENT consultant on call and list for rigid oesophagoscopy and foreign body removal

Q4. What signs and symptoms would make you concerned about a perforation?

Severe chest pain, tachycardia, tachypnoea, pyrexia, surgical emphysema, haematemesis

Q5. What would your management of a perforation be?

CXR, rigid oesophagoscopy, pass a nasogastric (NG) tube and leave in situ, confirm placement of NG, commence feed when happy in correct place

Lateral soft tissue neck (LSTN) X-rays can give very useful information in patients presenting with a history of a possible foreign body. Some foreign bodies are radio-opaque (including dentures, chicken bones and some fish bones including cod and haddock) and the LSTN can help localise it prior to removal. However, many foreign bodies are radiolucent (including some plastics and fish bones including mackerel, trout or pike) and therefore softer signs need to be utilised for diagnosis. These include loss of cervical lordosis, pre-vertebral soft tissue thickening and air in the oesophagus.

Physical examination should always include a close look +/− palpation of the tonsils as these are common places for foreign bodies to become embedded and can be easily removed in A&E or acute clinic. If no foreign bodies are found on oral examination, a nasendoscopy can be performed. If none are visualised but there are convincing clinical symptoms, a CT can help localise foreign bodies prior to panendoscopy and removal.

CASE 37

Q1. What is this?
Q2. When would you use it?
Q3. How does it work?

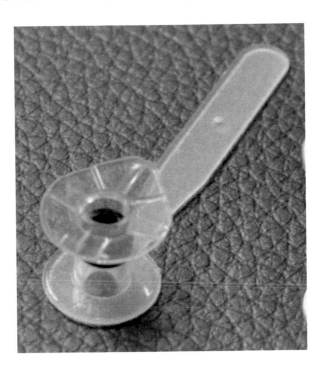

CASE 37 ANSWERS

Q1. What is this?

Blom-Singer valve (transoesophageal voice prosthesis)

Q2. When would you use it?

For speech production in laryngectomy patients

Q3. How does it work?

When the stoma is occluded, air is transmitted from the trachea into the oesophagus through the prosthesis and then through the throat which creates a voice sound. A small valve flaps back to prevent aspiration of food or liquids

Following laryngectomy, patients no longer have a connection from the lungs and trachea to the mouth. This means expired air does not cause vibrations of the vocal cords and cannot be articulated to produce speech. Multiple methods of voicing have been developed over the years. Computers can be used as speech synthesisers, or the remaining anatomy can be used to simulate speech.

Oesophageal speech is when swallowed air is regurgitated producing vibrations in the neopharynx that can be articulated by the tongue and lips. It is difficult to learn but can be very effective in some patients.

An electrolarynx is a handheld battery-operated device pressed against the skin of the upper neck that produces monotone buzz that the user articulates into speech. This is easy to use but creates a very 'robotic' voice quality that many patients dislike.

A trans-oesophageal puncture allows a one-way valve called trans-oesophageal prosthesis (TOP or TEP) to be inserted through the posterior tracheal wall into the oesophagus with a stabilising flange on either side. When the normal laryngectomy opening is occluded and the patient exhales, air is diverted through the prosthesis, up through the neopharynx into the oral cavity for articulation.

CASE 38

Q1. What is this?
Q2. What condition is it used in?
Q3. How does it work?

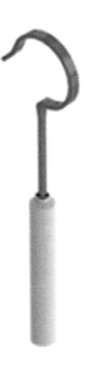

CASE 38 ANSWERS

Q1. What is this?

  Stapes prosthesis

Q2. What condition is it used in?

  Otosclerosis (inserted as part of a stapedectomy)

Q3. How does it work?

  The metal portion hooks around the incus and the other end is inserted through the stapes footplate to transmit sound vibrations to the inner ear.

Stapes surgery, commonly known as 'stapedectomy' is a treatment for otosclerosis and any other cause of stapes fixation. The middle ear is entered by lifting the tympanic membrane. The bony scutum may then be widened for greater access, aiming to preserve the chorda tympani which lie in the same plane. After confirmation of stapes fixation by testing ossicular chain mobility, then incudostapedial joint is divided. The stapedius tendon is then divided, followed by the posterior crus of the stapes suprastructure. The stapes suprastructure is then downfractured and removed. A hole is then made in the stapes footplate. Typically this might measure 0.4–0.6mm. Prosthesis is placed onto the long process of incus and passes through the footplate fenestration. This then restores the conduction of sound from the tympanic membrane all the way through to the inner ear. Risks to explain in the consent process include: dead ear, worsening or failure to improve hearing, infection, bleeding, dizziness, tinnitus, altered taste, facial palsy, perilymph leak, prosthesis failure and tympanic membrane perforation.

CASE 39

Q1. What is this?
Q2. Name one advantage over a grommet.
Q3. Name one disadvantage compared with a grommet.

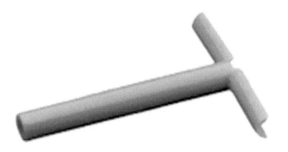

CASE 39 ANSWERS

Q1. What is this?

T Tube

Q2. Name one advantage over a grommet.

Remains in the tympanic membrane for longer

Q3. Name one disadvantage compared with a grommet.

Higher risk of residual tympanic perforation

T-tubes are used for chronic middle ear dysfunction which would otherwise necessitate the repeated insertion of conventional grommets. The aim is to permanently ventilate the middle ear space and prevent effusion and/or prevent progressive retraction of the tympanic membrane that may result in ossicular erosion and cholesteatoma. T-tubes are more commonly used in adults, for whom maturation of eustachian tube function (and therefore resolution of the need for a grommet) is not expected like it is in children. However, children with severely negative middle ear pressure leading to chronic disease may also benefit. T-tubes are associated with a higher tympanic membrane perforation rate compared to conventional grommets.

CASE 40

Q1. What is this?

Q2. What is the smallest of the above three components made from and why?

Q3. Name two situations where this would be more appropriate than a conventional hearing aid.

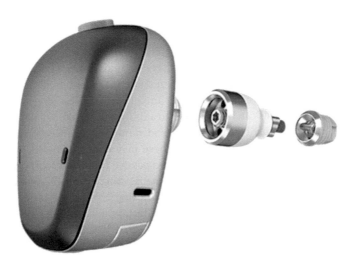

CASE 40 ANSWERS

Q1. What is this?

Bone anchored hearing aid

Q2. What is the smallest of the above three components made from and why?

Titanium as it osseointegrates

Q3. Name two situations where this would be more appropriate than a conventional hearing aid.

Congenital malformations of the middle or external ear, microtia, chronically discharging ear

A bone anchored hearing aid is a type of bone conduction device. These should be considered for any patient who is failing/unable to benefit from conventional hearing aids and yet has adequate cochlear reserve to benefit from amplification of sound.

Bone conduction devices can be divided into aids (which are often worn on a headband) and implants. Implants may be further subdivided into percutaneous (skin-penetrating) and transcutaneous (magnetic processor). These may even further be subdivided into active (powered component under the skin) and passive (powered component outside the skin). This is an ever-evolving field and audiometric criteria should be referred to for the latest available devices. Reasons for patients not being able to use conventional hearing aids include: recurrent infection, the occlusion effect, problems with feedback, unfavourable anatomy (e.g. microtia) and anxiety around stigma. Bone Conduction devices can also be used for patients with profound single sided deafness, by routing sound to the contralateral ear via bone conduction which has a very low attenuation across the skull.

CASE 41

Q1. What is the most common type of thyroid cancer?
Q2. Which thyroid cancer would give an elevated calcitonin level?
Q3. Which wider group of disorders is this type associated with?
Q4. What is typically the most aggressive form of thyroid cancer?
Q5. What is the primary investigation for a patient with a thyroid lump?
Q6. How would you proceed with a U4 Thy3f result and why?
Q7. How would you proceed with a Thy1 result and why?

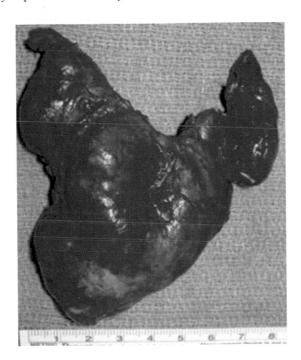

CASE 41 ANSWERS

Q1. What is the most common type of thyroid cancer?
    Papillary thyroid cancer

Q2. Which thyroid cancer would give an elevated calcitonin level?
    Medullary thyroid cancer

Q3. Which wider group of disorders is this type associated with?
    Multiple endocrine neoplasia type 2 (MEN2)

Q4. What is typically the most aggressive form of thyroid cancer?
    Anaplastic thyroid cancer

Q5. What is the primary investigation for a patient with a thyroid lump?
    Ultrasound and fine needle aspiration

Q6. How would you proceed with a U4 Thy3f result and why?
    Diagnostic hemithyroidectomy due to being unable to differentiate on cytology alone

Q7. How would you proceed with a Thy1 result and why?
    Repeat FNA as inadequate result

The thyroid parenchyma consists of follicular cells and the parafollicular or C-cells. Differentiated thyroid cancer includes follicular, Hurthle cell and papillary thyroid cancer. The parafollicular cells give rise to medullary thyroid carcinoma. Thyroid function tests should be requested for patients presenting with a thyroid nodule as patients with hyperthyroidism are less likely to have malignancy and a radionuclide uptake scan is indicated. In all other cases a thyroid ultrasound with FNA is indicated. Surgical excision remains the primary treatment of differentiated thyroid cancer with postoperative radioiodine ablation depending on the staging. Medullary thyroid cancer is treated by total thyroidectomy with neck dissection. Radioiodine is not used for medullary thyroid cancer given the distinction in embryological origin of it and differentiated thyroid cancer.

CASE 42

Q1. Describe object A.
Q2. What is object B and what is its use?
Q3. What is object C and what is its use?
Q4. Name four indications for tracheostomy insertion.
Q5. What is object D and how does it work?

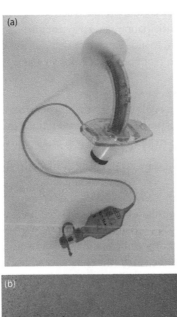

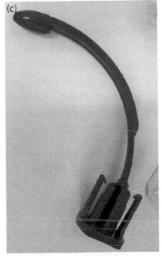

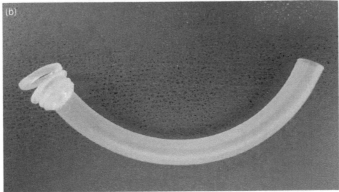

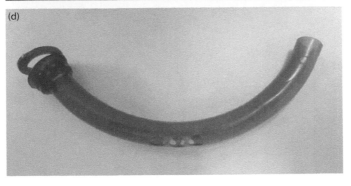

CASE 42 ANSWERS

Q1. Describe object A.

Cuffed fenestrated size 8 tracheostomy tube

Q2. What is object B and what is its use?

Non-fenestrated inner tube – to aid cleaning

Q3. What is object C and what is its use?

Introducer – to aid insertion of tracheostomy

Q4. Name four indications for tracheostomy insertion.

To secure an airway if compromised secondary to obstruction (infection/tumour/ trauma), to secure an airway in anticipation of airway compromise, to facilitate weaning for prolonged ventilation, to aid removal of respiratory secretions/ protect from aspiration, severe sleep apnoea not responsive to continuous positive airway pressure

Q5. What is object D and how does it work?

Fenestrated inner tube allows passage of air through the tracheostomy tube to the vocal cords allowing speech production. However, fenestrations can encourage granulation formation which leads to bleeding and potentially airway obstruction.

A tracheostomy is a surgical procedure whereby an opening is made in the anterior trachea in order to facilitate ventilation. Emergency tracheostomy is undertaken in the context of acute airway obstruction e.g. foreign body aspiration, Ludwig angina, obstructive laryngeal cancer, or where endotracheal intubation is not possible. Indications for elective tracheostomy include ventilatory wean, as a part of head and neck cancer treatment, subglottic stenosis and chronic aspiration. Early complications include bleeding, infection and pneumothorax. Late complications include subglottic stenosis and tracheoinnominate fistula (a rare but potentially life-threatening complication that presents with significant bleeding).

CASE 43

Q1. What clinical sign is this?

Q2. Which structure may be blocked to cause this symptom, and where does it open in the nasal cavity?

Q3. Name two acquired causes which may result in this symptom?

Q4. What endoscopic procedure can be performed to treat this condition?

Q5. Name two complications of this procedure.

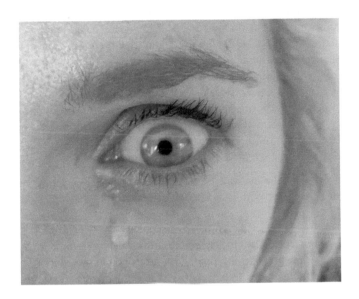

CASE 43 ANSWERS

Q1. What clinical sign is this?

Epiphora

Q2. Which structure may be blocked to cause this symptom, and where does it open in the nasal cavity?

Nasolacrimal duct, inferior meatus

Q3. Name two acquired causes which may result in this symptom?

Dacryocystits or nasolacrimal duct obstruction (NLDO): Chronic rhinosinusitis, impacted turbinate, previous FESS, dacryolithiasis, nasal orbital ethmoid fractures, neoplasms (lymphoma, SCC, inverting papilloma, sinonasal tumours), periorbital radiotherapy, some chemotherapy agents (docetaxel, paclitaxel, 5-fluorouracil), Radioactive iodine 131 therapy, inflammatory disease (sarcoidosis, granulomatosis with polyangiitis, Eosinophilic angiocentric fibrosis/IgG4-related disease), dental impaction

Q4. What endoscopic procedure can be performed to treat this condition?

Dacrocystorhinostomy (DCR)

Q5. Name two complications of this procedure.

Haemorrhage, orbital injury, infection, restenosis, adhesions.

Epiphora or tearing of the eye can be a complication of FESS if the nasolacrimal duct is damaged. It can be avoided by not extending the middle meatal antrostomy too far anteriorly.

Other causes include dacryocystitis or nasolacrimal duct obstruction. The nasolacrimal duct may be obstructed by blockage or strictures: dacryolithiasis, chronic rhinosinusitis, previous FESS, naso-orbito-ethmoidal fractures, neoplasms, periorbital radiotherapy, some chemotherapy agents or inflammatory disease (e.g. sarcoidosis or granulomatosis with polyangiitis).

Conservative methods for managing epiphora include massaging, compression and probing the nasolacrimal duct. If these methods fail, the patient may be offered an endoscopic dacrocystorhinostomy (DCR). This procedure involves endoscopically lifting a mucosal flap to identify the lacrimal bone and opening it to expose the lacrimal sac. The inferior canaliculus of the lower eyelid is then cannulated with a probe to confirm the location of the lacrimal sac and to tent the medial sac wall. The sac is then opened widely and a sialastic stent can be inserted along the path of the probe and secured in the nasal cavity.

CASE 44

Name the following oral conditions

Q1.

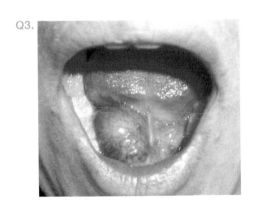

Q2.

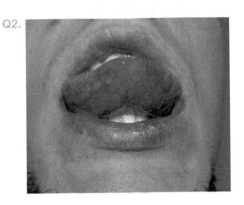

Q3.

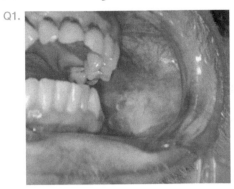

Q4.

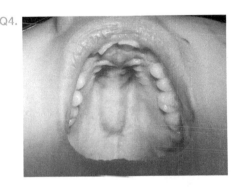

Q5.

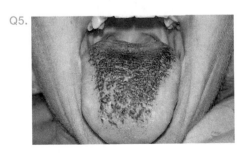

Q6.

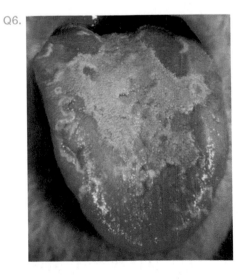

CASE 44 ANSWERS

Q1. Leukoplakia
Q2. Mucous retention cyst
Q3. Ranula
Q4. Maxillary torus
Q5. Black hairy tongue
Q6. Geographic tongue

ENT surgeons and GPs with a special interest in ENT often examine the mouth and it is very useful to have some knowledge of common oral lesions to be aware of. This article has an excellent summary with clinical images of lesions you may encounter, https://www1.racgp.org.au/ajgp/2020/september/common-benign-and-malignant-oral-mucosal-disease.

CASE 45

Q1. What type of imaging has been used to evaluate this patient?

Q2. Name two benefits and two disadvantages of this imaging modality.

Q3. What are the two main differential diagnoses for this patient?

Q4. Name three symptoms this patient is likely to experience.

Q5. Name the most important two components of the initial management of this patient.

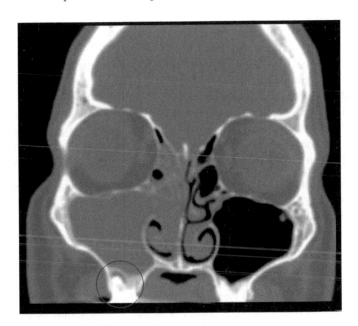

CASE 45 ANSWERS

Q1. What type of imaging has been used to evaluate this patient?

CT of the paranasal sinuses

Q2. Name two benefits and two disadvantages of this imaging modality.

Advantages: Painless, non-invasive, evaluate bony erosion/deformation, more information than OPG, quicker than MRI, helpful information for surgical planning (including for image guidance), can be performed with implanted medical devices.

Disadvantages: Radiation exposure; poor evaluation of soft tissues; expensive (compared to XR), patients must lie flat and still.

Q3. What are the two main differential diagnoses for this patient?

Fungal ball, tumour

Q4. Name three symptoms this patient is likely to experience.

Unilateral nasal obstruction; facial pain/pressure; foul odour/rotten taste; tooth pain

Q5. Name the most important two components of the initial management of this patient.

Medical management (antibiotics covering anaerobic bacteria) and dental extraction. (FESS is used when medical and dental treatment have been unsuccessful.)

Odontogenic sinusitis is diagnosed when sinonasal disease is thought to be of dental origin. Odontogenic sinusitis accounts for approximately 10% of sinusitis cases and is most common among 40–60 years old with a slight female predominance.

Dental procedures or periodontal/periapical disease in the maxillary molar teeth can breach the mucoperiosteum of the maxillary sinus (the Schneiderian membrane), which consequently impairs the mucocilary function and causes bacterial infection and inflammation.

Patients present with typical symptoms of sinusitis, with only a third reporting associated dental pain. A comprehensive history is required as there may be a latency of up to a year for dental surgery associated sinusitis or four years in implant-associated sinusitis. Anterior rhinoscopy may demonstrate unilateral mucopus or oedema. Oral examination may indicate the general state of the dentition and gums as well as oral-antral fistulas.

Orthopantomogram (OPG) can show periapical lesions, maxillary cysts and thickening along the floor of the maxillary sinus, with a sensitivity to detect dental cares and periodontal disease of 60%–85%. CT scans are more sensitive and will often show unilateral maxillary sinusitis as well as the dental source.

Odontogenic sinusitis infections are generally polymicrobial with predominantly anaerobic organisms, with highest susceptibility to piperacillin and co-amoxiclav with fluoroquinolones in penicillin allergic patients.

Treatment includes treating the dental cause (i.e. root canal, apicoectomy or dental extraction) in addition to medical therapy of systemic antibiotics, saline nasal irrigation and nasal steroid drops. If this does not control the symptoms, ESS may be required.

Index